MW00800025

Children with Autism Spectrum Disorders

Children with Autism Spectrum Disorders:

A Structured Teaching and Experience-Based Program for Therapists, Teachers, and Parents

Vera Bernard-Opitz

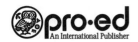
pro·ed
An International Publisher

8700 Shoal Creek Boulevard
Austin, Texas 78757-6897
800/897-3202
Fax 800/397-7633
www.proedinc.com

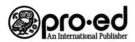

© 2007 by PRO-ED, Inc.
8700 Shoal Creek Boulevard
Austin, Texas 78757-6897
800/897-3202   Fax 800/397-7633
www.proedinc.com

All rights reserved. No part of the material protected by this
copyright notice may be reproduced or used in any form or by
any means, electronic or mechanical, including photocopying,
recording, or by any information storage and retrieval system,
without prior written permission of the copyright owner.

NOTICE: PRO-ED grants permission to the user of this book
to copy Appendix 5.A and Appendixes 7.A and 7.B for teaching
or clinical purposes. Duplication of this material for commercial
use is prohibited.

Originally published as *Kinder mit Autismus-Spektrum-Störungen*
(ASS): Ein Praxishandbuch für Therapeuten, Eltern und Lehrer,
© W. Kolhammer GmbH Stuttgart, Germany, 2005

Library of Congress Cataloging-in-Publication Data

Bernard-Opitz, Vera.
    [Kinder mit Autismus-Spektrum-Störungen (ASS). English]
Children with autism spectrum disorders : a structured teaching and experience-based
program for therapists, teachers, and parents / Vera Bernard-Opitz.
        p.   cm.
    Includes bibliographical references and index.
    ISBN-13: 978-1-4164-0232-9
    ISBN-10: 1-4164-0232-2
    1. Autism in children—Popular works.   2. Autistic children—Popular works.   I. Title.
RJ506.A9B3713   2007
618.92'85882—dc22

                                                                    2006024723

Art Director: Jason Crosier
Designer: Kim Worley
Illustrator: Andrea Bernard
This book is designed in FairfieldLH and Futura.

Printed in the United States of America

In memory of my parents,

Aute and Luzia Opitz

Contents

Preface

Knowledge about autism spectrum disorders (ASD) and effective treatment methods has increased significantly over the last 35 years. For the broad spectrum of impairments there are now evidence-based intervention methods. In the early 1970s, parents and professionals were usually helpless when confronted with the behavior problems of affected children, but we now have well-documented therapy options available.

Despite the advances, however, there is still a heated debate among some "therapy camps" regarding the most effective intervention. This treatment manual considers an integrated approach. Instead of assuming that one treatment fits all kinds of children with autism, I prescribe a continuum of methods, which is necessary for the heterogeneous group of children with ASD. The manual provides concrete examples of applied behavior analysis, precision teaching, experience-based interventions, and visual approaches in an integrated curriculum, called STEP, which has been used for more than 20 years.

The purpose of this book is to give parents and professionals an overview of structured interventions, helping them to be more successful and confident with their children with ASD. The STEP curriculum, which stands for *structured therapy and experience-based programs,* aims to help parents and professionals develop appropriate treatment goals and match intervention methods to the individual child. The book provides guidelines that will allow parents and professionals to predict which treatment may be more successful for a particular child. The last chapter is dedicated to parents and describes ways to set up a home therapy program. Throughout the book, I have supplied many concrete examples to make this manual as comprehensible and as practical as possible.

Consider this book as only a first step in teaching children with ASD. The STEP curriculum is not a static cookbook, but a set of flexible guidelines that need to be developed further through experience with children and increasing knowledge. As parents and professionals begin following the program, they can expect consistent but slow steps of progress for some children and big strides of development for others.

ACKNOWLEDGMENTS

Many colleagues, parents, and children have contributed in a direct or an indirect manner to this manual. First I want to thank my PhD supervisors, Erna Duhm and Friedrich Specht, both retired professors from the University of Göttingen, who instilled ideals about helping children with developmental delays and autism. I owe my behavioral background and interest in parent training and curriculum development to a large extent to Robert Koegel, University of California Santa Barbara, who supervised the applied part of my thesis. The late Carol Prutting, from the same university, has had an important influence on me and other colleagues. She always stressed linguistic and developmental approaches, and her kind ways will never be forgotten.

Over the years, many teaching ideas and intervention methods either have been developed independently or have been influenced by others. I am grateful for these ideas because they have significantly enriched the presented work. I especially want to acknowledge colleagues involved in applied behavior intervention, especially Ivar Lovaas, Catherine Maurice, Ron Leaf, and John McEachin; colleagues who shared their experience with precision teaching, such as David Leach, Michael Fabrizio, and Allyson Moore; colleagues who alerted us to communicative and play-oriented methods, such as Kathleen Ann Quill, Sabrina Freeman, Lorelei Dake, Adriana Schuler, and Pamela Wolfberg; colleagues involved in visual support systems, such as Lori Frost, Andy Bondy, and Linda Hodgon; and last, but not least, the incredibly helpful TEACCH team with Eric Schopler, Gary Mesibov, Ron Larson, and others.

I am also truly grateful to my long-term colleague Elizabeth McInnis of the Stein Center in San Diego. Over the past 25 years she and her excellent team of teachers have demonstrated that even severely challenged children with ASD can be helped through tireless efforts, using child-tailored training programs. My thanks go especially to Cheryl Armstrong, Mary McIntosh, Chris Gommel, and Barbara Almquist.

Upon return to my home country, Germany, I had the opportunity to establish a communication-training center for children, youth, and adults with ASD at the Johannes Rehabilitation Center in Mosbach. This constituted the first structured treatment program within a large German rehabilitation center. Our work was often difficult, but many residents benefited and developed alternatives to behavior problems and better means by which to communicate. I very much appreciate the support of the members of the Management and the Psychological Service, including Volker Dehn, Peter Rösinger, Günter and Werner Blesch, Ursula Müller-Dietrich, Karin Holz, Dünna Leib, and Julia Henkel.

I moved to Singapore and gained new experience and perspective. Through the help of Ann Devadas, first principal of Margaret Drive Special School, and a team of enthusiastic teachers, I developed the STEP curriculum, which involved more than 100 children over a 10-year period. S. Vasoo, former head of the Department of Social Work and Psychology of the National University of Singapore, supported a behavior intervention and autism research center at the university. During this period, the STEP curriculum was developed and applied to many children with ASD. This would not have been possible without my research assistants, especially Annabel Chen, Adrian Kok, Sharul Sapuan, Tan Yew Kong, Tan Yit Lai, Nah Yong Hwee, and Siow Ing. Many of the training programs described in this manual have been enriched through regular exchanges with Salwanizah Bte Mohd Said, the highly dedicated head of the Early Intervention Program of the Autistic Association Singapore.

Many colleagues have given highly valuable feedback to this book, such as Adriana Schuler, San Francisco; Gary Mesibov, TEACCH, Chapel Hill, N.C.; Titus McInnis, San Diego, Calif.; Charlotte Witsoe, Mission Viejo, Calif.; Evelyn Seika, Dubai, United Arab Emirates; Hanne Dirlich-Wilhelm, Munich, Germany; Fritz Poustka and Sven Bolte, Frankfurt, Germany; and especially my long-term colleagues and friends Ute Genser-Dittmann, Heidelberg, Germany, and Ann Devadas, Singapore. To Ute and Ann, I give a special thanks for all the long hours spent helping with translating, editing, and streamlining my manuscript.

Much appreciation goes to Chris Olson Becker for her superb help in preparing the manuscript. Thank you also to Courtney King and Chris Anne Worsham from PRO-ED, who have patiently accepted all last-minute changes. They have very much contributed to the new layout of this book, which was originally published in German by Kohlhammer under the good guidance of Ruprecht Poensgen. To all involved, a very honest thank you.

There is a long list of children and parents who have been partners in developing the STEP approach. I am grateful that many ideas we developed together now can be shared with others.

Last, but by no means least, I would like to express my gratitude to my family, who tolerated my long hours of typing when I could have been spending free time with them. They believed in my work and supported it in any way they could. My compliments to our children, Marian and Andra, for their technical help and for refreshing sketches. To my husband, Hans-Ulrich Bernard, I provide my deepest gratitude for his encouragement throughout this project.

Introduction

The incidence of infantile autism as a syndrome has increased significantly in the last 10 years. In 1968, the assumed rate of autism among children was about 4 in 10,000, but according to estimates by some autism experts, by the year 2000 this figure had increased 200% to more than 1 child with autism in 1,000. It is vigorously debated whether the observed increase is due to better and more systematic diagnosis or whether autistic disorders in fact have become more frequent (California Department of Developmental Services, 1999; Fombonne, 2003).

What are autism spectrum disorders (ASD) and how can they be treated most successfully? This guide addresses these questions from parents and therapists. The practical section of the book (Chapter 7) describes a behavioral training program developed specifically for young children exhibiting autistic behavior and associated problems such as attention-deficit disorders, hyperactivity, and learning difficulties.

The background section of this book (Chapters 1–6) is based on the latest international research in the field. Case examples are drawn from many years of experience with more than 1,000 children with ASD in early intervention programs, special schools, autism centers, rehabilitation centers, and a university clinic in locations as diverse as California, Germany, and Singapore. Empirically validated methods and curricula are presented concisely for easy reference.

Children with ASD display a wide variety of behavioral, motivational, and learning problems, which are not addressed satisfactorily by undifferentiated standardized therapies or single-track interventions claiming universal application. In contrast, this book demonstrates that successful therapy is a clearly structured, transparent process that is centered on the problems, interests, and abilities of the individual child. Specific suggested therapies are derived from a behavioral analysis and the child's skills. Examples in the book demonstrate that diagnostic observation and intervention must complement each other like key and lock.

This book compares treatment approaches that have been proven successful in helping children with autism and presents a curriculum with specific examples from acknowledged teaching methods. The reader will become familiar with a spectrum of methods from the traditional behavioral teaching format; precision teaching; experience-based teaching; and visual strategies like hand signing, the Picture Exchange Communication System (PECS; Frost & Brady, 1985), and the TEACCH program (Treatment and Education of Autistic and Related Communication-Handicapped Children; Mesibov, Shea, & Schopler, 2004). The included task sequences are designed to help parents and therapists plan training programs and carry them out in a structured manner. Specific guidance is provided for intensive training at home.

What Are Autism Spectrum Disorders?

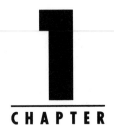

Chapter Overview

Definition of Autism Spectrum Disorders

Diagnosis of ASD

Early Signs of ASD

Factors Contributing to the Prognosis

Summary

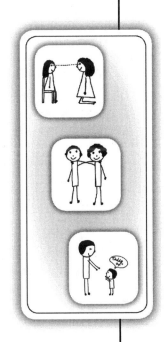

DEFINITION OF AUTISM SPECTRUM DISORDERS

Since infantile autism was first described by Leo Kanner in 1943 and Asperger in 1944, the diagnostic and therapeutic approaches have changed dramatically (Asperger, 1944; Kanner, 1943; Koegel et al., 1998; Lord & Schopler, 1994; Lovaas, 1968; Maurice, Green, & Luce, 1996; McEachin, Smith, & Lovaas, 1993; Prizant et al., 1997). Autism is now treated as a serious disorder that affects large areas of childhood development. As its name, *Autism Spectrum Disorders,* suggests, it represents a continuum of symptoms and degrees of severity (National Institute of Medical Health, 2004; Wing, 1988; Wing & Gould, 1979). The symptoms and the abilities profile range from severe impairment to almost normal behavior.

ASD are manifested differently from one child to another and their nature often changes in the same child as he or she develops. There is no single behavior that always occurs and no behavior that automatically precludes a diagnosis of autism. On the other hand, there are clear commonalities that are found in most people suffering from ASD, such as distinctive social behaviors (Committee on Educational Interventions, 2001). Perception disorders, communication features, deficits in social behavior, and intelligence vary widely among those affected, from barely perceptible disorders to severe impairment.

Just as the word *house* can mean an apartment block, a villa, or a log cabin, the term *autism* also has many variants. An individual with autism can live independently and pursue a profession as a tradesman, office worker, freelance artist, or academic, but at the other end of the scale, individuals with autism include those who are unable to speak, have never learned to care for themselves, and need assistance throughout their lives. At the same time—just like houses—people with autism also share a number of common features. The next section attempts to demonstrate these common features and corresponding interventions. Individual behavior problems, skills profiles, and interests must be matched to specific interventions just like a unique key only opens a very specific door.

The following box lists some of the disorders included in the autism spectrum.

Autism spectrum disorders include the following:

- Infantile autism
- Asperger's syndrome
- Rett's syndrome
- Disintegrative disorder
- Pervasive developmental disorder—not otherwise specified

For most continental Europeans, autism connotes *profound developmental disorders* (Dilling & Freyberger, 1999), but the Anglo-Saxon world has adopted the term *autism spectrum disorders.* ASD is a blanket description that encompasses not only childhood/infantile autism but also Asperger's syndrome, Rett's syndrome, disintegrative disorder, and nonspecific developmental problems or pervasive developmental disorder—not otherwise specified (American Psychiatric Association, 1994; National Institute of Mental Health, 2004). Infantile autism is viewed as a typical variant of ASD and is also known by the name *Kanner syndrome.* Asperger's syndrome, which was portrayed in the popular film *Rain Man,* is a milder variant of this. Cases of Rett's syndrome and disintegrative disorders in children are rare and for this reason are usually discussed separately. In this book, ASD will be understood to include childhood/infantile autism and Asperger's syndrome, which is the common usage. Many of the methods and exercises described also may be applied to children suffering from other profound development disorders, but would need to be adapted accordingly. In all cases, planning of treatments depends not so much on the specific diagnostic classification as on the individual child and his or her abilities and problems.

A specialized psychologist, psychiatrist, or neurologist must perform a comprehensive examination to differentiate ASD from similar disorders, such as depression; anxiety; hospitalism; encephalitis; infantile schizophrenia; Lesch-Nyan syndrome; Angelmann's syndrome; intellectual disability; or perceptual disorders, like auditory processing problems (Volkmar, Klin, & Cohen, 1997).

DIAGNOSIS OF ASD

The following list summarizes the diagnostic procedure in cases where autism is suspected.

Summary of Diagnostic Procedure for Suspected ASD

Is there evidence of an autistic disorder?
- Distinctive social behavior
- Communication and language features
- Repetitive and stereotypic behavior and desire for sameness

What is the child's developmental and intelligence level?
- Normal or delayed
- Special deficits and skills
- Intelligence profile

What additional problems exist?
- Physical characteristics (e.g., hearing, vision)
- Sleeping or eating disorders
- Attention-deficit disorder
- Sensory and motor problems

What are the early signs?
- Warning signs
- Prognosis
- Skills-oriented procedure
- Deficits and skills

What is the social environment like?
- Family history
- Social and cultural context
- Parenting style

The diagnostic procedure for suspected ASD is discussed in detail in the following sections.

Evidence of an Autistic Disorder

Autism disorders in children are diagnosed through observation and questionnaires. The *Checklist for Autism in Toddlers* (Baron-Cohen, Allen, & Gillberg, 1992) helps pinpoint symptoms of autism before the age of 18 months. General educators, nurses, and pediatricians also can use it as a method of gathering rough data. An autistic disorder can be suspected based on five behavior indicators, described below:

Indicators of Autistic Impairment in Infants

Questions to the Parents

- Does your child play imaginatively (e.g., does your child pretend to drive a toy car or to make tea with toy cups)?
- Does your child ever point to something interesting with her or his finger?

Direct Observation

- Does the child pretend to fly an airplane toy, to make a cup of tea, or play with other imaginative toys during the examination (e.g., flying, pouring, drinking)?
- Does the child follow the direction of your finger when you point to something interesting in the room (e.g., "Look, there's a spinning top")? Does she or he then look at the object or only at the pointing finger?
- Does the child look at you and at the object at which you are pointing (e.g., "Where's the teddy bear?")?

This abbreviated checklist indicates a risk of autistic impairment. If the key behaviors described above are not observed, the complete checklist should be administered a month later. The *Checklist for Autism in Toddlers* is not a diagnostic tool and must be supplemented with diagnostic procedures if autism is suspected.

The *Autism Diagnostic Interview Schedule–Revised* (Lord, Rutter, & Le Conteur, 1994) and its associated observation system, the *Autism Diagnostic Observation Schedule–Generic* (Di Lavore, Lord, & Rutter, 1995), are much more sophisticated. Clinicians must be specially trained to use these tools and have extensive experience diagnosing autistic disorders. These instruments help assess features of social interaction and play, such as making eye contact, smiling, pretending, imitating, making friends with peers, and interacting affectively with others. Another area of assessment relates to communication, such as pointing, nodding, shaking the head, using echolalic or functional language, or conversing. The third diagnostic area relates to repeated and stereotypical behavior and limited interests. A child's unusual preferences, compulsive routines, verbal rituals, stereotypical movements, and perceptual problems are investigated. Figure 1.1 summarizes the features assessed in the *Autism Diagnostic Interview Schedule–Revised*.

Michael, 5 years old, spent most of his time dangling objects and opening and closing doors. If interrupted, he would scream for long periods and could not be calmed.

The development of Rosa, 18 years old, was significantly impaired by severe compulsive and self-injuring behaviors. She banged her head against surfaces so hard that she had to receive stitches on several occasions. Although she had only a mild learning disability, she was considered unteachable because her behavioral disorders were severely compulsive. She did not mind receiving negative conse-

Diagnosis of Autism

Social interaction and play

- Making eye contact
- Smiling
- Pretending
- Imitating
- Making friends

Communication

- Pointing
- Nodding, shaking head
- Using echolalic or functional language
- Conversing

Repeated behavior and limited interests

- Unusual interests and preferences
- Rituals, stereotypical movements
- Perceptual problems

FIGURE 1.1. Summary of behavior characteristics assessed using the *Autism Diagnostic Interview Schedule–Revised* (Lord, Rutter, & Le Conteur, 1994).

quences to her behavior as long as the consequences were predictable. Therefore, we began providing unpredictable consequences to her behavior. This turn of events was highly effective in reducing the self-injurious behaviors.

Perceptual disorders and compulsive behaviors can also be observed in people with ASD and normal intelligence. The following example shows that from the point of view of the person affected, behavior problems serve a clear function.

A laboratory assistant with ASD would lock herself in the bathroom at work several times a day. Inside, she would jump up and down and hit herself because her body felt numb.

Some children tear their clothes off because they cannot stand the feeling of the fabric on their skin or the label in the back of a T-shirt. Others are so insensitive to pain that even a broken finger can go undiscovered for quite a long time. Others refuse to eat solid food or certain types of food, while their counterparts will eat inedible objects. Extreme hypersensitivity and hyposensitivity can also be observed with smells. Some children sniff at objects that have no odor, while others seem to find the normal world of smells unbearable. Autobiographical reports indicate that inconsistency can occur within different perceptual channels. The same sound may be perceived as too soft on one occasion and unbearably loud shortly thereafter (Grandin & Scariano, 1986; White & White, 1987; Williams, 1992).

Communication problems often are noticed as the first indicators of autism. Only half the children at the lower end of the autism spectrum are capable of functional speech. At the higher end of the spectrum, pedantic speech, monologues, and disregard for the interest and prerequisite knowledge of the listener are obvious.

The behavior of children with ASD is not always as noticeable as in the examples provided earlier. The problems of those at the higher end of the spectrum are often much more subtle and relate to impaired awareness of others, social behavior, and independence. Those problems require targeted therapy too.

After several years of intensive therapy, 10-year-old Mathew appeared to have been "cured." However, his parents reported the following incident: One day, Mathew vanished without a trace from a party held in the community. After searching without success for a long time, his parents called the police. The police finally found the boy asleep in his own bed. Mathew explained that he had gone home because it was dark and he always went to bed when it got dark.

Mathew obviously lacked the ability to understand that his parents would be concerned if he did not tell them where he was going. His only concern was to follow the rule he knew: "When it's dark, it's time to go to bed."

Developmental and Intelligence Levels

Generally, the developmental and intelligence levels of a child with ASD can be seen as a skills profile with positive and negative sides. Often children with ASD have good visual–spatial skills but perform poorly on language-related tasks. Good treatment plans need to raise the developmental level and balance the individual skills profile with its associated strengths and weaknesses.

Infantile autism is generally ranked as the most extreme of autism spectrum disorders, because in 75% to 80% of cases, it is characterized by significantly lowered intelligence. At the other end of the scale, children with Asperger's syndrome usually have normal or above-average intelligence (American Psychiatric Association, 1994). Often, a distinction is made between high-functioning and low-functioning children with autism (Perry & Condillac, 2003), which reflects above- or below-average IQ. Therapy programs for both groups are generally quite different. Therapy with low-functioning children concentrates on establishing eye contact, imitating, sorting, communicating simply, and playing, whereas teachers of high-functioning children need to emphasize social behaviors, emotional intelligence, independence, and self-control, in addition to helping with specific learning difficulties.

The following factors are keys to testing the intelligence of children with ASD:

- Use motivating tasks
- Make procedures visual
- Test for brief periods

These techniques are discussed in more detail below.

When assessing a child's developmental and intelligence levels, the clinician must ensure that assessment tasks are motivating and presented in a way that suits the child. Accordingly, the selection of more appropriate tests or the adaptation of conventional tests has enabled some children who were originally considered to be untestable to achieve age-appropriate nonverbal intelligence scores.

When testing children with infantile autism, the clinician often must rely on visual, non–language-based procedures such as the *Leiter International Performance Scale* (Roid & Miller, 1997) or the *Progressive Matrices* (Raven, 2004). For such instruments, the child must insert or fit blocks or cards showing different colors, shapes, symbols, or pictures in the correct slots.

Traditional intelligence tests sometimes can be adapted slightly to fit the learning needs of individual children. For example, some children achieved appropriate scores in the popular Wechsler test series only when the testing periods were kept short and the trials were presented visually, not just verbally (Kaufman, 1994). Getting social or material reinforcement for their efforts, not for correct answers, also enhanced performance.

Scales that help assess an individual's independence and adaptive skills, such as the *Vineland Adaptive Behavior Scales* (Sparrow, Balla, & Cicchetti, 1984), should also be used with children with ASD. These instruments are helpful for establishing a realistic assessment of self-sufficiency in areas like daily living skills, socialization, and play or leisure time. This area is often neglected, particularly for children with Asperger's syndrome or infantile autism and high intelligence.

Additional Problems

Most children with ASD suffer from nonspecific neurological problems (Bölte & Poustka, 2002a). Even if no specific organic problems are found, epileptic seizures are an ever-present danger. One in six children with ASD experiences such attacks during puberty (Gillberg, 1990). The degree to which the child is affected and the effectiveness of the medication used to control the seizures have a significant bearing on the child's prognosis.

The clinician should explore other potential problems, such as depression, anxiety and sleep disorders, attention-deficit/hyperactivity disorder, sensory–motor problems, Tourette's syndrome, and compulsive behaviors, during the first meetings with a child's parents. Children with Asperger's syndrome are more prone to depression and anxiety attacks than a comparable group of typical children (Perry & Condillac, 2003). Some children with these disorders can be helped with medication (Bölte & Poustka, 2002b) in addition to behavioral therapy. For example, the medication Risperdal has been shown to be effective with children exhibiting aggressive, anxious, or compulsive behaviors (McDougle et al., 1998).

Sleep disorders also can be treated both with behavioral therapy and medication (Durand, 1998). Melatonin has been described recently as an effective sleep inducer for children with ASD. New medications like Adderal, Concerta, or Stratera have been shown effective for attention-deficit disorders, and they cause fewer side effects and last longer than commonly prescribed stimulants such as Ritalin or Cylert. Behavioral training programs for improving attention and learning in children with attention-deficit disorder also offer some help for children with ASD who have similar difficulties (Barkley, 2006).

About half of all children with ASD suffer from impaired hearing, impaired vision, or sensory–motor abnormalities (Ayres, 1979; Frith & Baron-Cohen, 1987; Myles et al., 2000). Vestibular problems are obvious in children who frequently spin, jump, or climb. Others react anxiously if their position changes or if balance is required. These children clearly resist being lifted into the air, spun around, or even rocked.

Reports from individuals with ASD indicate that abnormal perceptions can cause behavioral difficulties (Grandin & Scariano, 1986; White & White, 1987). For example, simply shaking hands with someone with ASD can be painful when that person is unaware that his or her hand squeezes the other too hard.

These problems are often addressed with occupational, speech and language, sensory–motor, or auditory integration therapy (Ayres, 1979; Berard, 1993; Myles et al., 2000). Sensory integration therapies evaluate children for sensory processing problems and provide the children with appropriate stimulation, such as touch or practice with balance. Sensory integration therapy seems a logical approach to addressing the multitude of sensory–motor problems of children with ASD, while attempts to improve a child's auditory processes through listening programs with filtered music also seem to make sense. Programs directed at auditory or sensory–motor problems have had strong support from parents and well-meaning professionals, even without sufficient evidence of the effectiveness of these treatments.

The few existing objective outcome studies on sensory integration therapy had few participants and lacked a control condition. One of the studies with a larger sample and a counterbalanced design did not support sensory integration. It found that children vocalized better during tabletop activities, rather than in sensory activities. (For a review, see Dawson & Watling, 2000.)

Empirical studies of auditory integration therapy have had a similar result. Four of the five outcome studies did not support the positive claims of the proponents. One study found greater improvement in the auditory integration therapy group compared to the control group, but this study had methodological difficulties (Dawson & Watling, 2000). One study revealed no difference in the behavior of children who had listened to unfiltered music compared to those who had listened to music with filtered frequencies (Bettison, 1996). Parents and professionals, therefore, should bear in mind that presently there is no scientific research confirming the effectiveness of sensory integration therapy or auditory integration therapy in reducing problem behaviors or increasing desired behaviors in children with ASD (Dawson & Watling, 2000; Committee on Educational Interventions, 2001; Shaw, 2002).

On the other hand, the lack of empirical data does not demonstrate that a treatment is ineffective (Committee on Educational Interventions, 2001). To evaluate treatment effects, clinicians may need to match treatments to the specific needs of individual children (Schreibman & Koegel, 2005). Well-controlled comparison research and individualized treatments are highly needed, especially when problems in areas such as sensory–motor development are obvious in the ASD population.

EARLY SIGNS OF ASD

Typically developing infants make eye contact and smile by the time they are 3 months old; these first communications are not evident in infants with autistic behaviors. Troubling signs may appear in some children even in the first year of life, such as failure to follow a person with their eyes, failure to search for the source of surprising or frightening situations, inattention when a partner points to something, and failure to make gestures. One of the earliest indications that an infant may be suffering from autism is that she or he does not make pointing gestures, particularly failing to point to draw attention to something, called *proto-declarative pointing*. Some children do point, but they use the gesture only when they want something, called *proto-imperative pointing* (Mundy, Sigman, & Kasari, 1994).

Many parents report that their child "lives in his [or her] own little world" and is emotionally self-contained, laughing or crying for no apparent reason. Some children even cry inconsolably for hours for no obvious reason. Lack of interest in adults or other children, failure to imitate or speak, and the absence of normal play are frequent signs that prompt parents to contact a specialist. According to its definition, an autistic disability can be expected to appear before the age of 36 months (American Psychiatric Association, 1994). Difficulties become most apparent between the ages of 3 and 5 years (Klicpera, Bormann-Kischkel, & Gasteiger-Klicpera, 2001). The following box summarizes early warning signs.

Early Warning Signs for ASD

Problems with

- eye tracking
- pointing
- imaginative play
- language development
- communication

FACTORS CONTRIBUTING TO THE PROGNOSIS

The prognosis for a child exhibiting autistic behavior depends critically on the severity of symptoms and expected response to treatment. Other crucial factors include what the child's developmental level is; whether he or she develops functional language skills by the age of 5 years; whether organic problems such as a seizure disorder are present; and what the child's therapeutic, schooling, and family circumstances are. The prognosis is generally considered favorable in cases of mild autistic disorders among children with normal intelligence and functional language skills who receive support from therapists, teachers, and family members, and undergo intensive training between the ages of 2 years and 4 years (Howlin, 1997). Retrospective video recordings have shown that children for whom the prognosis was good demonstrated spontaneous speech on the earliest recordings, unlike the children for whom the prognosis was less optimistic (Prizant & Wetherby, 1998). Recently joint attention and symbolic play have been demonstrated as positive predictors for later language development (Kasari, 2004).

But even if these optimal circumstances are not in place, the clinician should focus not on the child's weaknesses, but rather on his or her skills and incorporating them into the training program. For example, the clinician should note that a child solves complex puzzles, imitates gestures, says two words, and smiles at a person playing peekaboo rather than compile endless lists of what she or he cannot do. The latter serves only to discourage everyone concerned. In addition, the clinician should help parents think positively because it seems important for the prognosis (Durand, 2004). The following box lists some of the factors that may influence a child's prognosis.

Factors Affecting Prognosis

Autistic behavior

- Nature and severity of problems
- Treatability

Special deficits and skills

- Developmental level
- Language skills before age of 5 years
- Sensory disorders
- Motivation and interests

(continues)

Organic problems
- Nature and severity of problems
- Treatability

Family and training options
- Optimism
- Training possibilities
- Financial situation

ROLE OF THE SOCIAL ENVIRONMENT

To get a more complete picture of a child with autism, a clinician also must consider family history and the social environment. Parents should be asked about the age, sibling position, and development of their other children and possible developmental difficulties in their own history (Lord, Rutter, & Le Couteur, 1994). Caregiver arrangements and experience with schooling and treatments also should be investigated. Asking parents to describe a typical day in their child's life often is very informative.

Cultural contexts and socioeconomic levels also constitute crucial components of the assessment because behavior abnormalities are viewed in different ways by different groups and access to educational services and treatment can be affected by poverty level and ethnicity. In addition, early interaction patterns between infants and their caregivers differ significantly across ethnic groups and among children with different educational and economic backgrounds (Brown & Rogers, 2003).

Even though a majority of studies has ruled out that social class or race is a risk factor for autism (Fombonne, 2003), information on the cultural, economic, and educational background of the family and on languages used is important so that support and treatment can be matched to specific family settings. I have met Singaporean children with ASD who have been exposed to up to four languages, with the parents speaking Mandarin, the grandparents conversing in a dialect, the caregiver from the Phillipines speaking Tagaloc, and schools using English. Some of these children seemed most comfortable with games and books on ABCs and 123s because everyone said those in English. Clearly, sensitivity to the child's individual social environment is highly important.

Coping and parenting styles are also crucial factors in the child's day-to-day experience. While research indicates that most families cope well (Harris, 1994), mothers of children with ASD report more stress in their lives than mothers of children with other developmental disabilities (Rodrigue, Morgan, & Geffken, 1990). Some parents handle their children with authoritarian parenting styles, expecting obedience and respect for authority. Others are more willing to negotiate, valuing their children's individualism. These styles interact with cultural values and need to be carefully considered when matching treatment not only to the child but also to the context of his or her family (Brown & Rogers, 2003).

SUMMARY

Autism spectrum disorders encompass a continuum of behavioral problems that vary widely in nature, severity, and prognosis. Diagnosis of an autistic disorder is based on questionnaires and observation. The prognosis and therapy planning depend in large part on an understanding of the behavioral problems and the creation of an intelligence and skills profile. Infantile autism often occurs in conjunction with other problems, such as attention, perceptual, or sleep disorders. In some cases, medication can be beneficial in addition to structured and sensory–motor therapies. A positive attitude toward their child on the part of parents can also have a positive influence on the prognosis. In addition to focusing on the child, the assessment should shed light on his or her social, economic, and linguistic context. Treatment methods need to be matched not only to the child, but also to his or her environment.

Therapy Approaches

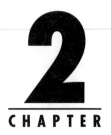

Chapter Overview

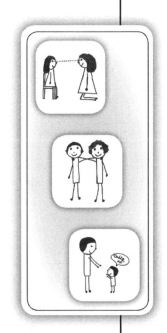

For many years, children diagnosed with infantile autism were classified as incurable. Only about 5% of these children could expect close-to-normal development; the vast majority lived in institutions for the mentally handicapped. Today, due to the availability of effective interventions (Graff, Green, & Libby, 1998), the prognosis is less bleak.

Is There a Universal Treatment?

Since autism was first described in the 1940s, therapies from a broad spectrum have claimed positive outcomes or even recovery from autism. Methods as diverse as facilitated communication (Biklen, 1993), holding therapy (Welsch, 1989), and auditory integration training (Berard, 1993) have given hope to parents. Unfortunately for most families this hope was short-lived because these methods were unsubstantiated by objective data (Gravel, 1994; Prior & Cummins, 1992; Shane, 1994).

One of the core assumptions of the above proponents was that *all* children with ASD could benefit from or possibly even be cured through one of those interventions. Some therapists thought that a trusting relationship was the key to the world of the autistic child, while others believed sensory–motor therapies, music therapies, or specialized diets were universally beneficial. Unfortunately, most proponents of these approaches failed to demonstrate their effectiveness in independent, well-controlled studies, and parents found it very difficult to make good choices for their children (Mastergeorge, Rogers, Corbett, & Solomon, 2003).

We know today that autism spectrum disorders constitute a highly heterogeneous group that requires complex evaluation, not simple answers. There is no question that a trusting relationship between child and therapist is an important component of successful learning, but this alone is not sufficient. Even for therapies as widespread as sensorimotor intervention, there is only limited empirical support regarding beneficial effects for the overall group of children with ASD (Baranek, 2002; Siegel, 2003).

Because approaches such as these have not been objectively substantiated, parents and clinicians should share the responsibility of determining whether individual features of affected children justify participation in controlled trial treatments (Howlin, 1997). To make informed decisions, parents and clinicians should consider critical reviews by reputable organizations and an independent evaluation of these approaches by experienced researchers (e.g., Association for Science in Autism Treatment, http://www.asatonline.org). Even though best-practice guidelines specifying safeguards have been suggested for some of the untraditional methods such as facilitated communication, clinicians should consider the ramifications of losing valuable time in children's education, disappointing parents through claims of a cure-all, and wasting money and other resources (Schopler & Mesibov, 1994).

Presently, the vast majority of research studies concentrate on behavioral interventions, structured teaching systems, and developmental therapies, all of which have demonstrated their effectiveness in sound research studies over the last 40 years.

Applied Behavior Analysis and Its Influence on Therapy

Applied behavior analysis (ABA) is the application of behavioral principles to the understanding and modifying of behavior. It is traditionally defined as "... the science in which procedures derived from the principles of behavior are systematically applied to improve socially significant behavior to a meaningful degree and to demonstrate empirically the procedures employed were responsible for the improvement in behavior" (Baer, Wolf, & Risley, 1968). ABA is rooted in learning theory and stresses that antecedents and consequences determine behavior. Antecedents can be defined as events that happen before the behavior occurs, while consequences are the events that happen immediately following the behavior. For example, a child who is praised or rewarded for greeting appropriately is more likely to greet again than if she or he is ignored or berated.

Discrete Trial Format

ABA, as a learning theory, can be seen in a variety of therapy methods, the most traditional being the *discrete trial format*. Promoted by Ivar Lovaas (1968), discrete trial format involves small therapeutic steps with clear and repeated instructions. Following a correct response from the child, the therapist administers a direct consequence. With this technique, Lovaas was able to reinforce the basic skills, such as imitation and language, in children with ASD; he also was able to reduce the severity of these children's behavioral problems (R. Koegel, Russo, & Rincover, 1977). Unfortunately, longitudinal analyses showed that the discrete trial format yielded poor spontaneity and weak generalization for many children (R. Koegel & Koegel, 1988).

Natural Language Paradigm

To address the problems associated with discrete trial format, several of Lovaas' students developed the *natural language paradigm* (Laski, Charlop, & Schreibman, 1988). The natural language paradigm emphasizes the child's initiative, seeks to use natural reinforcers, which are consequences directly related to the behavior, and encourages generalization of mastered skills. A child who is allowed to go outside after saying, "Bye-bye" is more likely to use and generalize this word compared with a child who repeats this word in a table setting and is reinforced with a food item. Teaching is transferred from the clinic to the everyday environment with the child's interest serving as a starting point for interventions.

Pivotal Response Training

By the end of the 1980s, *pivotal response training* (Koegel & Koegel, 1988; Koegel, 1999) developed as a new ABA therapy, drawing on both discrete trial format and natural language paradigm. This approach concentrates primarily on building off pivotal behavior such as the child's motivation or initiative. For example, it has been shown that children who are allowed to choose tasks and who are reinforced for attempting to communicate are more motivated to learn (R. Koegel, O'Dell, & Dunlap, 1988; R. Koegel & Williams, 1980). A child who is allowed to use the bubble wand for approximating the word *bubble* is more likely to repeat this word as compared to a child who is required to say the whole word correctly before being allowed to use the wand.

Precision Teaching

Independently of these other approaches, Lindsley (1964, 1972) had developed *precision teaching* during the 1960s. In this program, small therapy steps are practiced for short periods of time, from 10 to 60 seconds, until they become automatic. For example, a child who cannot read, write, or count quickly enough will have difficulty with more complex tasks such as problem solving. The objective of precision teaching is to ensure that skills such as imitating, reading, and basic arithmetic can be performed automatically and do not hinder the more complex tasks.

Over the last 40 years the repertoire of ABA methods has significantly evolved; some proponents claim that even "Dr. Lovaas doesn't do Lovaas Therapy any more" (Leaf, 1998). Besides the described discrete trial format (Koegel, Rincover, & Egel, 1982; Maurice et al., 1996) and the natural language paradigm (Laski et al., 1988), pivotal response training (Koegel & Frea, 1993; Koegel & Kern-Koegel, 2005), verbal behavior (Sundberg & Partington, 1999), and precision teaching (Fabrizio & Ferris, 2003; Lindsley, 1964) are now considered under the ABA umbrella. Over the years, ABA has been increasingly conducted in more natural environments, with a loosened structure and more frequent opportunities for children to initiate and to engage in social interaction with their peers.

STRUCTURED TEACHING

As mentioned, many programs for children with ASD are based on applied behavior analysis, but two other foundational approaches exist: *structured teaching* and *developmental approaches*, which follow developmental patterns in typical children (also referred to as *social–pragmatic*). Parents and professionals frequently associate ABA with the discrete trial format promoted by Lovaas and associate structured teaching with the TEACCH program (Treatment and Education for Autistic and Related Communication Handicapped Children) developed by Eric Schopler (Schopler & Mesibov, 1994; Schopler, Mesibov, & Shea, 2004).

In North Carolina, at about the same time as advances in the discrete trial format occurred, Schopler was developing the *TEACCH Program*. The main features of the program include learning in a structured environment with clear expectations and schedules, and receiving early encouragement for independence. The learning situation is visual, with unambiguous task structures, pictures, symbols, and activity schedules. Visual boundaries are created using partitions or tape on the floor, which assist the child with ASD in differentiating various activities. Personalized work systems are developed to help children understand what is expected and to ensure the development of independent work habits.

Like ABA, structured teaching programs have also diversified over the years, and proponents have become more interested in obtaining systematic measures of progress. The focus of the TEACCH program on visually structured tasks and environment has given rise to programs such as the *Picture Exchange Communication System* (Frost & Bondy, 2002), *picture activity schedules* (Hodgdon, 2000; McClannahan & Krantz, 1999), and *social stories* (Gray, 2004). The good visual capability of many children with ASD has also been the basis for the development of visual communication systems such as *sign language training*. These methods will be described in detail in the next chapter.

EXPERIENCE-BASED THERAPY

In addition to the above interventions, there is mounting evidence for the effectiveness of methods stressing the child's experience as well as social, pragmatic, and developmental aspects, such as *activity-based instruction* (Pretti-Frontczak & Bricker, 2004), *social–pragmatic developmental approaches* (Prizant & Wetherby, 1998; Prizant et al., 2005), and *integrated play groups* (Schuler & Wolfberg, 2000).

Concentration on experience, activities, and social relationships has achieved a new importance, particularly with the advent of new findings in the fields of developmental linguistics and emotional learning (Twachtman-Cullen, 2004). Linguists have shown that comprehension is an important prerequisite for developing meaningful expression in children with ASD. This can be enhanced through play and daily activities (Schuler & Wolfberg, 2000). Emotional experiences, such as excitement, joy, and fear, facilitate learning and retention (Wolfe & Brandt, 1998). Experience- and activity-based instructions have a naturalistic teaching approach. Important premises are that the children have to experience things for themselves and the therapists are required to establish a good relationship as the foundation for learning. Over time, this highly diverse conglomeration of ideas has evolved into a series of concrete programs with clear therapy sequences (Gutstein & Sheely, 2002).

EVIDENCE-BASED PRACTICES

In recent years, the term *evidence-based practices* has become a buzz phrase used to indicate treatments that have passed empirical tests, thus demonstrating their quality, effectiveness, and usefulness (American Psychological Association, 2002). How effective are intensive ABA programs, play-oriented methods, the Picture Exchange Communication System, the TEACCH program, or social stories? Parents and professionals need to know whether a method has been tested and whether the risks of wasting time, energy, and money, or of raising false hopes, outweigh the benefits (Perry & Condillac, 2003). Obviously, there are different levels of evidence, such as anecdotal evidence, controlled-group designs, and single-subject designs. Anecdotal evidence alone is not sufficient, but controlled-group designs and replicated single-subject designs can validate treatment. The intervention methods included in this manual are those backed by rigorous, scientific research that produces consistent findings no matter how many times the study is repeated.

Even though there are clear differences in schools of thought and practice for all of the above methods, there is considerable overlap. In the early years, ABA, structured teaching, and developmental methods were considered to be incompatible with each other. Over the last 15 years, however, there has been a shift, and behavior intervention is no longer viewed as a process by which individuals are changed to the environment, but rather one in which the environment can be adapted to individual needs, sometimes also described as *positive behavior support* (Horner et al., 2000). While proponents of this approach have had a significant influence on therapeutic and educational practices, more traditional behavioral methods are still required for children with more need for structure (Prizant & Wetherby, 1998; Sundberg & Partington, 1999). Mounting evidence shows that children with ASD constitute a spectrum of various skill profiles and learning needs. These needs must be matched to specific interventions that have proven effective with groups of similar children. The question is no longer, "Which method is best?" but "Which method is best for which child, and which therapy goal should be targeted?" The first research in this area is on its way, demonstrating that behavioral and play interventions affect behavior characteristics of children with ASD in highly specific ways (Bernard-Opitz, Ing, & Tan, 2004; Kok, Bernard-Opitz, & Tan, 2002). Treatment packages such as pivotal response training are also undergoing investigation for their most crucial components (Sherer & Schreibman, 2005).

THE STEP APPROACH

In 1988, my colleagues and I developed the Structured Teaching for Exceptional Pupils (STEP) program, which was the precursor to the curriculum presented in Chapter 7. The program began with 7 children, but quickly grew to more than 100 children with ASD (Bernard-Opitz, 1993). It had a clear structure of tasks and sequences and a well-defined basis in behavioral therapy. Visual support through hand signs and picture systems and adaptation to the child's preferred learning channel also were part of the program (Bernard-Opitz, Blesch, & Holz, 1988, 1992; Bernard-Opitz, 1983). The program also included experience-based, development-oriented, and motivational components. Emotional learning such as experiencing the sensations of surprise, joy, and mild stress was integrated systematically in individual programs. The STEP curriculum was a main part of the program, which was developed over the course of many years at the STEP program, incorporated in three locations: the Behavior Intervention Center for Children at the National University of Singapore; a rehabilitation center near Heidelberg, Germany (Johannes-Anstalten); and the Los Niños Center in San Diego, Calif. Excerpts from the curriculum are presented in Chapter 7.

In this manual we use the term *structured teaching and experience-based programs* (STEP) as a blanket term for effective therapeutic interventions that (a) have an empirical basis and a clear structure, (b) are directly related to the problems of children with autism, and (c) incorporate provisions for experience-based learning and individual, flexible planning (Bernard-Opitz, 1981, 1993; Mesibov, Schopler, & Hearsay, 1994). STEP may be seen as a continuum of therapy options that include key strategies for children with autism, matching individual features and specific intervention methods.

SUMMARY

In the last 40 years a continuum of evidence-based intervention approaches has been successfully used with children with ASD (Hoagwood et al., 2001; Prizant & Wetherby, 1998). Unlike the holistic therapeutic approaches, applied behavior analysis, structured therapies, and developmentally based interventions have an empirical basis and are directly related to the problems of children with ASD. Many diverse methods have evolved from the origins of traditional discrete trial learning and structured teaching methods. Natural, experience-based learning, training in key behavior strategies, and time-based and visual programs were introduced in this chapter. They are integrated in the STEP curriculum presented in the second half of this book. Specifics about the mentioned interventions can be found in the following chapter.

Therapies for Children with Autism Spectrum Disorders

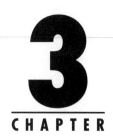

3
CHAPTER

Chapter Overview

Components of STEP

Usefulness of STEP Methods

What Is the Success of the STEP Methods?

Summary

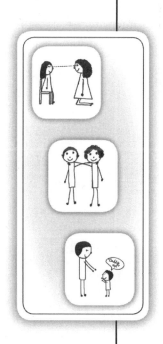

Therapy approaches for people with autism should include a variety of methods that address the full spectrum of the disorder. The STEP (Structured Teaching and Experience-based Program) presented in Chapter 7 in this manual combines evidence-based best practices from several teaching methods introduced in the previous chapter: discrete trial training, precision teaching, experience-based learning, and visual strategies. The various methods are matched to the individual learning features of children with ASD. These methods will be explained in more detail throughout this chapter.

STEP Methods for the Treatment of ASD

Traditional Behavioral Methods

- Discrete trial format (R. Koegel, Russo, & Rincover, 1977; Leaf & McEachin, 1999; Lovaas, 1968; Maurice, Green, & Luce, 1996)
- Precision teaching (Leach et al., 2003; Lindsley, 1964, 1972)

Experience-Based Learning Methods

- Natural language paradigm (Laski et al., 1988)
- Pivotal response training (R. Koegel, 1999)
- Emotional/activity/play-based learning (Gutstein & Sheely, 2002; Prizant et al., 2005; Schuler & Wolfberg, 2000; Twachtman-Cullen, 2004)

Visual Approaches

- Hand-sign training
- Picture Exchange Communication System (PECS; Frost & Bondy, 2002)
- Pictured activity schedules (Hodgdon, 2000; McClannahan & Krantz, 1999)
- TEACCH program (Schopler & Mesibov, 1994; Schopler et al., 2004)

Although all of these methods are advocated as ways to teach children and adults with ASD, research comparing them is rare. While each method is backed by empirical data, none of the treatments has been clearly demonstrated to be superior to the others (Bernard-Opitz et al., 2004; Dawson & Osterling, 1997; Prizant & Wetherby, 1998). Consequently, STEP incorporates several evidence-based procedures and matches them to specific variables of children with ASD.

COMPONENTS OF STEP

The following summary demonstrates the features of STEP methods:

Discrete Trial Format
- Uses small teaching steps
- Involves mainly the trainer's initiative

- Makes use of discriminative stimuli, prompts, and reinforcement
- Involves repeated drills

Precision Teaching

- Uses small teaching steps
- Stresses rate of responding in small time units
- Uses the various input and output channels
- Assesses progress with standard celeration charts

Experience-Based Learning

- Emphasizes learning through experiences
- Involves incidental teaching
- Creates opportunities and relevant experiences
- Makes use of the child's initiative and spontaneity
- Involves interruption of everyday activity sequences

Visual Programs

- Use visual aids
- Use small and meaningful teaching steps
- Provide visual support through task structures and work systems
- Make use of the child's initiative and spontaneity

Discrete Trial Format

The discrete trial format is at the heart of intensive behavioral therapy programs for young children with autism. Described as discrete because it includes clearly separate components, the discrete trial involves the three basic elements of behavioral therapy: a stimulus, a behavioral response, and its reinforcing consequences.

A discrete trial format drill begins with a clearly defined task and is taught in the following way:

1. The therapist starts a trial with an instruction, called the *discriminative stimulus* (S-D). Examples of such stimuli are "Match," "What is this?" "What is mommy doing?" "Do you want this?" "Do this."
2. The child *responds* correctly or incorrectly, and receives the corresponding *consequence* from the therapist.

   - If the child answers correctly within about 3 seconds, he or she is praised and receives a preselected reinforcer, such as a small piece of candy, a toy, a hug, or something similar.
   - If the child does not respond or responds incorrectly, he or she is prompted to get it right.
   - The teacher's first choice of prompt should be the least restrictive one, which is *pointing*.
   - The next is a *distance prompt,* then *errorless prompt,* and finally *physical guidance.* Prompts must be effective and then faded over successive trials.

In the following example of the discrete trial format, the task is for the child to match two blue items with one distracter present.

Instruction	Response	Help (Prompt)	Consequence
"Match"	Child matches correctly.		"Good, that is (blue)." Child receives a raisin.
"Match"	Child makes incorrect choice.	Correct color is moved closer to the child. (Distance prompt)	Praise when prompted response is correct.

Levels of prompts should change according to the needs of each child. The goal is to provide the lowest level of prompting that prevents him or her from making the wrong response. Prompts should be chosen with consideration to the child's response type. A child with good visual skills is likely to respond to visual cues such as pointing, while another child may need full physical guidance to be successful. Prompts are classified according to the hierarchy below:

Prompt	Level	Example
Pointing prompt	Least restrictive	The therapist points to the correct object.
Distance prompt		The correct object is moved closer to the child.
Errorless prompt		The distracter (for example, a second sorting tray) is removed so that the child has only one color to match. In other words, the chances of making an error are reduced.
Physical guidance	Most restrictive	The child's hand is guided to the correct color.

Important elements of the discrete trial format

- Drills must be carried out repeatedly for children to achieve success. In general, at least 10 trials of each task are done per session.
- For a child to learn a discrimination task, such as matching the colors red and blue, the right–left position of the colored objects must be altered. This ensures that the child is responding to the objects and not to their position.
- To make discrimination easier in a standard teaching interaction, the therapist can present objects or instructions repeatedly. That is, the therapist gives one particular instruction five times before changing it. For example, the therapist might say, "Throw the ball" five times before changing the task slightly to "Throw the Frisbee." When the child has successfully made this discrimination, the number of repetitions can be reduced from five to three. Thus, the therapist asks the child three times to get the ball, and then three times to get the Frisbee. Finally, the trainer indicates the objects randomly. (A reproducible data recording form is provided in Appendix 7.B.)
- Steps in teaching are small, and each therapy target is used as the basis for the next. For example, imitating gross-motor actions is usually trained before copying fine-motor movements, followed by imitating sounds, and later, imitating words (Lovaas, 1981).
- As a rule, 8 correct responses in 10 attempts on two consecutive days are considered an adequate criterion for advancing to the next therapy step.

Some parents and therapists have difficulty coming to terms with the drill-like training of the discrete trial format. However, some more challenged children may need this method to learn effectively, and its primary purpose should be to create the conditions for less stringent approaches.

Shaping

Another important feature of behavioral interventions used in STEP is *shaping*. With this strategy, progressively closer approximations to the target behavior are taught. For example, a child who learns to imitate sounds initially receives a reinforcer for each sound he or she produces within 3 seconds following the model sound produced by the therapist. Over the course of consecutive trials, imitations must become more similar to the target sound before reinforcers are given.

Chaining

Chaining is another important part of the discrete trial method. Behaviors are broken into simple, manageable steps for children to learn. These small steps are taught sequentially as links in a chain.

In *forward chains*, the steps are taught from first to last. For example, the forward chain of teaching a child to eat ice cream independently might begin with the child picking up a spoon and eventually end with placing the spoon of ice cream in his or her mouth.

To teach this behavior as a *backward chain*, the therapist would teach the steps from last to first. The child would start by learning to put the spoon of ice cream into her or his mouth. The child then works backward, gradually doing more and more without any adult assistance. The last step would be to pick up the spoon. Backward chains are often more motivating than forward chains because the final reward—a mouthful of ice cream—is nearly always guaranteed.

Precision Teaching

Precision teaching is a method developed at Harvard University by Ogden Lindsley (1972) in the 1960s, and it grew out of the tradition of behaviorism. This approach was first tested in a Montessori class for children with learning difficulties. It has been used successfully with university graduates as well as students with severe intellectual disabilities (White, 1986).

Precision teaching is also called *fluency learning* because it stresses automatic, effortless performance. It is based on the assumption that the rate of responding—and not just the number of trials alone—is crucial for generalization (Kubina et al., 2002). The method is characterized by small, basic therapy steps, which must be attained within short time periods of 10, 20, 30, or 60 seconds. Children in programs for precision teaching are pressed for time and highly motivated. "How many action cards, opposite cards, or days of the week can I label within 20 or 30 seconds? Can I do better than last time?" Children learn to set their own timer and monitor their progress on standard celeration charts, which reflect the child's performance in specific time units. In general, a weekly goal is to double the frequency of a behavior after 1 week of fluency practice within the selected time unit (Johnson & Street, 2004). Teaching sessions should be carried out several times a day so that the learned response becomes automatic (Pennypacker, Koenig, & Lindsley, 1972; White & Haring, 1981).

Conducting Precision Teaching

In an example of precision teaching being used to develop legible handwriting, the student draws slashes, semicircles, or circles in various directions for periods of 20 seconds (Vargas & Vargas, 1991). The goal is to ensure that the child reaches automaticity when forming pencil strokes before he or she attempts to master the more complex task of forming letters. Performance standards are based on the frequency of correct responses during the first 10 trials. The child receives a token, such as a sticker, star, or smiley face, for each improvement.

Children who have a certain level of self-control may award themselves tokens. If a child has improved his or her performance at least three times, she or he receives a reinforcer previously agreed upon, like food or jumping on the trampoline. At a more advanced stage, children are taught to achieve preset goals, such as answering 30 questions about the calendar in 1 minute. They enter the number of correctly and incorrectly answered questions on paper logarithmic learning graphs and try to improve their answering rate every day until they reach the predetermined standard.

The most successful classes have been those in which the children take responsibility for their learning. They measure their own progress and plot their own learning curves. They decide with their teachers when and how the curriculum objectives can best be reached. This self-controlled learning is an important feature of precision teaching. (A reproducible data recording form is provided in Appendix 7.B.)

Generalization of Precision Teaching

When using precision teaching techniques, the therapist needs to confirm that the skills learned are generalized to nontaught settings and occur automatically in different learning channels. To accomplish this, children learn target behavior in various perceptual channels and modes of expression. For example, the activity of playing ball can involve the child imitating visual impressions (see–do): The child sees the ball rolling and rolls it back. But imitation can also involve repeating sounds and words (hear–say): The child hears the word "ball" and repeats it. A modified learning objective is that of naming the ball when it is seen or felt (see–say or feel–say) or perhaps also picking it out from among other objects when the word "ball" is heard (hear–do/show/give/touch; Fabrizio & Moors, 2003). For many children with ASD, the leap from visual differentiation to linguistic comprehension and expression is enormous and requires targeted training programs.

Examples follow of input and output channels being used in imitation and language exercises when playing with a ball:

Target Area	Input–Output	Therapist Instruction	Example
Imitation of movements with objects	See–do	"Do this." Therapist rolls the ball.	Child sees the ball rolling toward him or her and rolls it back.
Imitation of words	Hear–say	Therapist instructs, "Say *ball*."	Child hears the word "ball" and is instructed to say it.
Expressive communication	See–say	Therapist shows the ball and asks, "What is this?"	Child sees the ball and is instructed to name it.
Receptive communication	Hear–do (show, give, take, play)	Therapist instructs, "Show (or give or take) the ball."	Child is instructed to pick the ball out of a group of objects and point to it (or give it).

Natural Language Paradigm, Experience-Based Learning, and Play

As described in the previous chapter, Koegel, Schreibman, and colleagues, practicing the traditional behavioral therapy procedure, realized that even after intensive therapy many children demonstrated learned behavior only when asked to do so and did not transfer their skill to unstructured situations. In response to this, the natural language paradigm was developed with a special emphasis on children's spontaneity (R. Koegel et al., 1998). In this approach, behavioral methods are combined with other interventions derived from developmental psychology and speech therapy (Prizant & Wetherby, 1998; Prizant et al., 2005). One of these methods is called *interrupting behavior chains.* (A reproducible data recording form is provided in Appendix 7.B.)

Interrupting Behavior Chains

Speech therapy researchers (Goetz, Gee, & Sailor, 1985) noted that children communicated more spontaneously if they were interrupted during activities such as climbing stairs, eating, playing, or swinging. In studies, children were asked to make eye contact, say words, and recite the days of the week and even multiplication tables. This method of interrupting behavior chains often leads to increased attention and rapid learning, even among children with severe disabilities.

The following examples show how interrupting behavior chains works.

A child who likes to play basketball is interrupted whenever the ball falls through the net. He gets the ball back only when some form of communication is observed, which could be when the child makes eye contact, vocalizes, passes a photo of a ball to the interaction partner, or imitates a gesture. See Figure 3.1.

A child who loves soap bubbles is interrupted at various points of play, such as when she takes the top off the container, takes out the bubble wand, starts to blow, or tries to catch the bubbles. For this procedure to succeed, the therapist must attract the child's attention without causing frustration.

In the above examples, the child's own initiative and natural reinforcers are crucial.

Pivotal Response Training

The above methods were further developed in *pivotal response training* (R. Koegel & Koegel, 1988). In addition to the above-mentioned natural reinforcers, choosing between tasks, mixing easy and difficult tasks, and reinforcing attempts to communicate resulted in faster

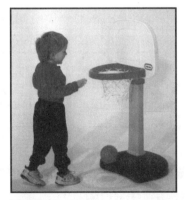

FIGURE 3.1. After every toss, the ball is withheld until the child looks at the interaction partner. (Source: *Picture This* Photo CD [2003], www.silverliningmm.com)

learning (R. Koegel, 1999). Some methods used to enhance the child's motivation are summarized below.

Motivation Enhancers

- A choice of tasks provided to child
- Mixture of simple and difficult tasks
- Reinforcement of steps in the right direction
- Natural reinforcers (i.e., ones that are related to the task)
- Interruption of behavior chains occurring in everyday activities
- Multiple examples of items used in targeted tasks
- Encouragement of child's interaction with teaching materials

In both the discrete trial format and pivotal response interactions, the child has to attend to the therapist or the task. She or he receives a clear instruction that is appropriate to the task. Unlike the discrete trial format, instructions in natural teaching interactions can be varied depending on the comprehension of the individual child. Variations link known words to unfamiliar ones so that a child learns concepts instead of specific object or action labels. Approximations of the child's response to the target behavior are reinforced, such as nodding or making a sound as communication for "yes." Natural reinforcers are used whenever possible, such as in the following example.

As Justin rolls cars down the ramp, his teacher says, "Vroom. Here comes the car ... another one." Before a car hits the gate, the teacher asks, "What do you want?" If Justin replies, "Open/the gate/please" or makes approximations, the teacher opens the gate and lets the car pass. After repeating this interaction a couple of times, the teacher switches roles with Justin and rolls other cars down the ramp (Teacher: "Vroom. Here comes the bus. Ask the bus driver: 'What do you want?'" Justin: "Open the gate"). The teacher may then encourage other play activities involving the bus, such as children getting on the bus to go to school.

In the above example, language and play are used multiple times, which allows generalization from the start (R. Koegel, 1999). For example, the child learns to name different kinds of vehicles (e.g., taxi, truck, bus), instead of working only on the word *car*. Similarly, after starting with models such as "open gate," the child can generalize to other things that also open, such as "open door."

Children tend to be more motivated when they can make choices and when they can be successful by performing easily mastered tasks, such as in the following example (Bernard-Opitz, 1985).

The behavior of 10-year-old Sui became considerably less confrontational when her therapist allowed her to select the task sequence and prompted her to demonstrate previously mastered tasks, such as counting on her fingers.

Differences Between the Discrete Trial Format and Natural Teaching Interactions

There are several distinct differences between the strategies of discrete trial teaching and natural language paradigm/pivotal response training. In discrete trials, the therapist begins a drill, decides on the exercises and materials, and uses simple and repetitive instructions such as "Give ...." Conversely, in the natural language paradigm and pivotal response training, the child initiates the learning process and the therapist takes his or her lead from whatever the child's interests are at the time. In this teaching format, the therapist's instructions often vary between drills to make sure the child is exposed to a range of commands. Approximations to the target behavior, such as sounds, are reinforced instead of the desired and appropriate verbal utterance. In the discrete trial format, consequences tend to be reinforcements unrelated to the target behavior, such as food when the child has copied building a tower with blocks. By contrast, in the natural learning methods, the consequence of a correct response tends to be a natural reinforcer, such as letting the child knock down the tower once she or he has built it. The following table summarizes some of these differences between the two methods.

Differences Between the Discrete Trial Format and the Natural Language Paradigm/Pivotal Response Training

Features	Discrete Trial Format	Natural Language Paradigm and Pivotal Response Training
Initiative	Teacher	Child
Instruction	Simple, repetitive	Flexible
Help device (prompt)	Special hierarchy	Flexible
Consequence	Artificial	Natural

As mentioned in the previous chapter, there were, at one time, heated debates between the proponents of traditional treatments (often referred to as "Lovaas therapies") and those of the new approaches described here, but over time many advocates of the two camps have grown steadily closer. Even the main proponents of traditional behavioral therapy approaches have begun to include aspects of speech therapy and developmental psychology in their training programs, so now it is truly possible to speak of a continuum, rather than a series, of separate treatment methods (Prizant & Wetherby, 1998).

Experience-Based Learning and Emotional Learning

As a result of this paradigm shift, there is now more tolerance for methods promoting *experience-based learning*, sometimes also associated with *emotional learning*. These approaches assert that the child should first gain some hands-on experience with instructional materials and only then can she or he assimilate and organize new concepts. The claim that hands-on experience is necessary is supported by evidence from the study of normal child development (Pretti-Frontczak & Bricker, 2004). Before a typical child learns a concept, she or he grasps it, literally. For example, a child puts a toy car in her or his mouth, feels it, turns its wheels, pushes it along different surfaces, and finally learns it will roll. Then there is the joy of finding out where it rolls slowly and where it rolls fast and discovering that it has similarities with daddy's car. All this is later associated with the word *car*. Being able to solve one's own problems and feel competent is a crucial component of self-initiated learning as practiced in the TEACCH program (Schopler et al., 2004).

Often a single experience is sufficient to recall important things. A child who has burnt his or her mouth eating soup will generally react more quickly to the word *hot* than one who has not yet done so. Many of us can remember experiences that are associated with emotions, even many years later, such as nervousness on the first day of school, a first kiss, the panic following news of an accident involving a loved one, or what we were doing when we first heard about the events of Sept. 11, 2001, in the United States. This rapid, emotional learning, which persists in a child's memory, can be useful, particularly for children who have difficulty learning normally. Children who participate in fun or trust exercises, such as jumping into the arms of an adult, tend to be more reliant on the adult than if the therapy situation were unpleasant (Gutstein & Sheely, 2002; Twachtman-Cullen, 2004).

Everyday experiences, such as learning what an apple feels or tastes like, trying on a shoe that is too big or too small, realizing that when something gets broken it can be repaired, form the basis for concept and language development among typical children. Learning that takes place when behavior is associated with natural consequences is generally more successful than learning that occurs through arbitrary consequences. The child who is told to "*Eat* the big cookie"—where there is a choice of two sizes—will be more motivated to differentiate between the sizes than the child who only is told to "*Point* to the big cookie."

The *mild stress method* can be used in many situations to motivate children to communicate appropriately. Even children with severe disabilities usually protest very quickly if they find themselves being coaxed into ill-fitting shoes or pants that are too large. Similarly, if a mother and child always make a right turn to catch the bus, and Mom suddenly takes a different route, the child will most certainly react and be very likely to communicate his protest. However, there are usually few motivation problems when children are offered several socks and told to put on a matching pair before going out to play (see Figure 3.2).

There are numerous other experiences that can stimulate problem solving and communication. A child must ask someone for help if he or she has been given a ball that has no air in it. It is not possible to obey an instruction to sit on a chair if there is no chair available; and what would you do if you found a hammer in the breadbasket or beside the plate instead of the breakfast you were expecting (see Figure 3.3)?

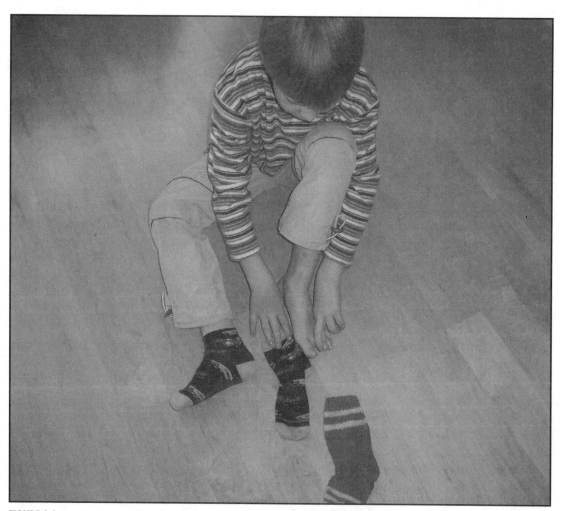

FIGURE 3.2. Daily activities such as dressing provide opportunities for learning colors, shapes, materials, and sizes.

Play is one of the activities and shared experiences typical children enjoy most. For children with ASD, however, playing with toys and engaging in peer play does not come naturally. As in many other areas of development, special methods of intervention are needed to help them catch up with their peers. Not only does facilitation of play enhance play skills and peer interaction, it also has a positive effect on language development. Recent research has demonstrated that children with autism between the ages of 3 and 5 years improved their verbal communication "just" through training of play and joint attention (Kasari, 2004).

Playing with peers has been stressed as an effective way of teaching children with ASD since the early 1990s. Initiated by Pamela Wolfberg and Adriana Schuler, *integrated playgroups* have been conducted for children with ASD and their siblings or peers. Studies have shown that children acquire communicative and social skills while playing with others (Kasari, 2004; Schuler & Wolfberg, 2000). They learn to imagine, solve problems, and negotiate with their peers while having fun and developing crucial friendships (Wolfberg, 2003; Yang et al., 2003). In integrated playgroups, small groups of children regularly play together while an experienced adult facilitates. Over a period of 6 to 12 months, the adult enhances the children's initiations and guides social and communicative exchanges. As the children with ASD improve, the so-called novice players and expert players develop more understanding and empathy (Wolfberg, 2003).

Visual Systems

Normal social interaction, communication, and play all require the ability to distinguish between what is important and what is not, and to respond quickly to various stimuli (Hodgdon,

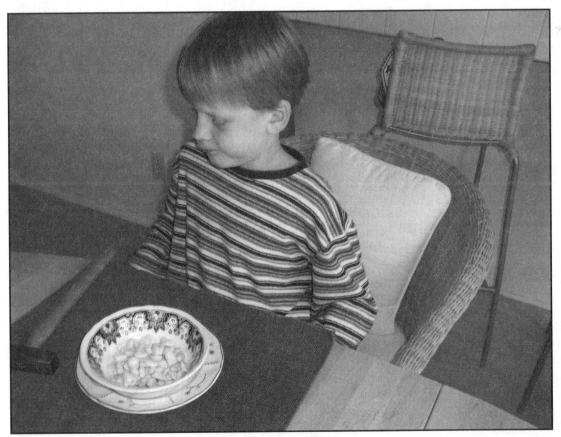

FIGURE 3.3. Unexpected settings make good triggers for attention and communication.

2000). Research and clinical experience indicate that children with ASD benefit from visual support and structure (Schopler et al., 2004). While they are often severely impaired in language and organizational systems, their visual–spatial skills frequently are good or even exceptional (Schopler et al., 2004). Inadequate processing of language and impairment in filtering out nonrelevant stimuli make it necessary to provide visual communication systems and unambiguous task structures.

Many children with ASD do not talk and do not respond appropriately to complex language, subtle facial expressions, or gestures. They tend to be overwhelmed by rapid speech and dynamic movements. In comparison, static communication modes, such as pictures, word cards, or to some extent even hand signs, are frequently more successful because they require slower visual processing and fit perfectly with the good visual abilities of this group of children. The table below shows perception differences between several communication methods.

Requirements for Different Communication Methods

	Learning Channel		Level of Consistency	
	Hearing	*Seeing*	*Dynamic*	*Static*
Language	✓		✓	
Facial expression		✓	✓	
Hand sign		✓	✓*	✓
Pictures		✓		✓
Word cards/Writing		✓		✓

*Hand signs vary in their dynamics.

Alternatives to language-based communication in the form of *word cards* were suggested for older, nonverbal children with autism as early as 1977 (LaVigna, 1977). A year later, *hand signs* were used successfully with children with ASD (Carr et al., 1978), and 10 years after that, children with autism in Germany learned to use either hand signs, word cards, or a picture communication system (Bernard-Opitz et al., 1988).

Picture Exchange Communication System

In the same period, the *Picture Exchange Communication System* (PECS; Frost & Bondy, 1985) was developed. In this program, children initiate communication by presenting pictures of their preferred items to their interaction partner in order; the children then receive the pictured objects. Compared with hand signs, PECS requires less complex motor movements. The system is relatively easy to teach, and children often show rapid learning rates. In many countries, nonverbal and beginning-verbal children with ASD now are equipped with PECS boards or PECS books, which help them to communicate requests or make descriptive utterances by handing single pictures or sentence strips from their PECS book to their partners (Charlop-Christy et al., 2002). Figure 3.4 shows a PECS board.

TEACCH Program

The *TEACCH* program (Schopler & Mesibov, 1994; Schopler et al., 2004) is based on the neuropsychological differences in children with ASD, such as their need for predictable situations and their good visual capabilities. Teaching targets are tailored to individual needs and are developmentally appropriate and meaningful. Tasks have a clear visual structure that indicates what to do, how to do it, and when the task is finished. The program promotes visual support

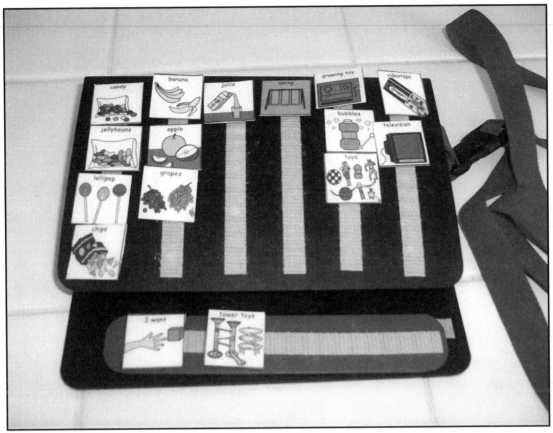

FIGURE 3.4. Children with good visual skills can communicate better through visual support systems, such as the *Picture Exchange Communication System* (PECS). (Source: www.pecs.com)

through a clearly structured environment, such as having the teacher create lines on the floor, color-code walls, define areas of the room, structure tasks clearly, and label activity areas and activity sequences, to serve as an orientation aid. Illustrated or written plans can be used to create a clear structure for the day, the sequence of events and exercises, or even the components of individual tasks. Pictured activity schedules help children visualize the daily order or task steps, such as the routine for washing hands or the steps involved in setting the table (Hodgdon, 2000; McClannahan & Krantz, 1999).

In the TEACCH method, tasks must be functional, worked through from left to right, and, once learned, generalized using similar materials. "Finish boxes" indicate that tasks have a definite end. The completion of tasks is therefore one of the main reinforcers in the TEACCH program. Figure 3.5 shows how a work area might be arranged under the TEACCH program. (A reproducible data recording form is provided in Appendix 7.B.)

USEFULNESS OF STEP METHODS

In the next chapter, the described traditional behavioral, experience-based, and visual methods will be combined under the blanket term "structured teaching and experience-based program" (STEP). The following list shows how STEP methods customize teaching for the individual learner.

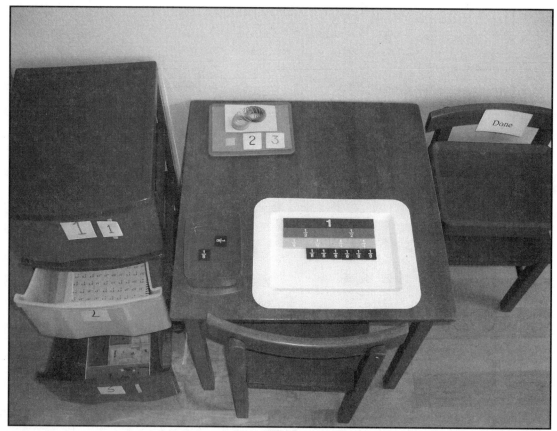

FIGURE 3.5. In the TEACCH program, clear task setups depict what needs to be done in what sequence.

STEP methods are matched to the features of learners with ASD

Attention, learning, and motivation problems

- Functional teaching targets
- Structured environments and tasks
- Well-sequenced tasks
- Short task duration
- Repetitive trials
- Powerful reinforcers
- Emotional and experience-based learning
- Enjoyable teaching interactions

Processing style

- Consideration of learning channels
- Visual support through pictures, word cards, symbols, hand signs
- Structured teaching environment, tasks, schedules

Insistence on sameness

- Predictable environments and learning settings
- Routine-based learning
- Scripted interactions

The following text explains how the features above match the needs of children with ASD:

- **Attention, learning, and motivation problems** are frequent in children with ASD, which can be overcome by instructional methods that focus on functional teaching targets, small teaching units, and powerful reinforcers.
- **Functional teaching targets** (i.e., those that are meaningful to a child) are more likely to be learned and generalized than those that are unrelated to the child's daily experience. Therefore, tasks such as learning prepositions presented in a table setting (e.g., Therapist: "Put the block over/under/behind the cup") result in nonattentive or confused children and, once learned, are not always generalized to other settings. On the other hand, tasks that provide relevant experience, such as, "Sit in/on/behind the toybox," make them more interesting to children. Once a child realizes that understanding prepositions matters and that his favorite balloon can be found either *behind* or *under* the sofa, the child's attention and enthusiasm increase.
- **Structured environments,** such as clear physical boundaries for the learning setting, reduce children's confusion. Visual schedules and **clearly organized tasks** help children with ASD understand what happens when and what is expected (Schopler et al., 2004).
- Children may also benefit from **well-sequenced brief tasks.** Because attention spans of 10, 20, and 30 seconds are manageable, fluency drills are often motivating. Children may practice labeling coins, telling time, or recalling simple math facts in these short periods. In addition, the tasks enhance learning and facilitate spontaneity and generalization.
- In the beginning of therapy, **repetitive trials** are frequently necessary to facilitate learning. Parents need to know that the first steps of learning are the hardest, sometimes requiring up to several hundred trials. Parents should know that learning gets easier with each successful step.
- Because many children with ASD fail to respond to subtle social cues, such as praise, it is often necessary to use **powerful reinforcers,** such as tangible goodies and sensory or natural reinforcement.
- Learning can be a chore or **an enjoyable experience.** If a child is asked to point 10 times to objects selected randomly by the therapist, she may wonder why. A child is more likely to stay motivated when pointing is associated with activities like poking bubbles or switching on the television remote control.
- **Learning channels** should be considered for all children, but especially for children with ASD because they process information differently. Children who have **problems processing** auditory cues, such as language and dynamic stimuli, need stable visual structures to learn effectively. Visual supports can include pictures, word cards, symbols, and hand signs. Children with autism who see on their visual schedule, for example, which tasks and events come next are calm and less irritable.
- Because **most children with ASD like stability** and dislike changes or surprises, interventions should be predictable, routine, or scripted.

Overall, teachers often see increased learning rates and a reduction of behavior problems when the teaching strategies that are used match their students' needs.

What Is the Success of STEP Methods?

The success of STEP methods has been demonstrated in many scientific publications. The Pub Med database alone lists more than 500 publications under "Autism and Behavior Therapy" dated after the mid-1960s. The following programs in particular have dominated the field of research: the early intervention program by Lovaas and his colleagues at the University of

California, Los Angeles (Lovaas, 1987; McEachin et al., 1993), the PECS by Frost and Bondy (2002), and the TEACCH program by Schopler and Mesibov (1994). While precision teaching has good empirical evidence for children with dyslexia and attention-deficit/hyperactivity disorder, support for children with ASD has only recently been demonstrated (Kubina et al., 2002; Simmons et al., 1998). Consider the following list, which exemplifies the success of STEP methods:

- Many scientific publications have confirmed the effectiveness of behavioral methods.
- Through intensive early intervention, children with ASD have made significant gains in all areas of development.
- The TEACCH method has been spread to autism programs around the world. Individuals from more than 45 states and 20 foreign countries have participated in TEACCH training activities (see http://www.teacch.com/aboutus.htm).
- Children in the precision teaching program at Morningside Academy in Seattle, Wash., tend to make 2 years' worth of progress in school-related tests after 1 year (Johnson & Street, 2004). Since 1991, the Morningside Teachers' Academy has successfully implemented precision teaching in 86 schools with more than 17,000 students throughout the United States.

Support for the Discrete Trial Format

In the intensive discrete trial format program, young children with autism involved 40 hours per week over 2 years made significant gains compared to children involved in a less intensive intervention of 10 hours per week. In his widely cited outcome study, Lovaas (1987) showed that 47% of 3- to 4-year-olds were successfully integrated into regular classrooms. At the age of 13 years, eight of the nine especially successful children of the intensive early intervention program were rated comparable in their IQs and their adaptive behaviors to their regular peers (McEachin et al., 1993). Unfortunately this optimistic picture has not been confirmed in follow-up studies, which have indicated success rates below 30% (see Shea, 2004).

While replication studies have not managed to attain the original success rates, they all have confirmed the positive effects of behavioral intervention (discrete trial format). In a pilot study with eight young autistic children, my colleagues and I investigated the effect of behavior and play interventions on the children. In as few as 10 weeks of structured training involving students and parents, we saw clear improvements in compliance, play, and communication. Five of the eight participants gained an average of 8.1 months on the *Symbolic Play Test* (Lowe & Costello, 1988), and seven of the children even reduced their score on the *Autism Diagnostic Observation Schedule* (Bernard-Opitz et al., 2004; Lord et al., 1994). Six of the eight children showed higher compliance and skill enhancement during the behavior condition in comparison to the play condition while two of the children improved in the play condition.

Based on these and other findings, one can expect that a discussion regarding the best treatment methods has to be refined to the question of which method works best with which teaching target for which child. More research is needed to understand how the specific characteristics of the children, the parents, and the therapists, and the specific teaching procedures, contribute to the overall outcome (Gresham & MacMillan, 1998).

Support for Precision Teaching

Empirical support for precision teaching with ASD populations is still not widely available. Ongoing research projects at various universities, anecdotal case reports, and observations by my colleagues and me show precision teaching as a promising intervention. Children with autism seem more attentive, react faster, and learn better when working on small teaching steps in short time intervals (Fabrizio & Moors, 2003; Kubina et al., 2002).

Presently there is more research evidence for precision teaching as used with children with attention-deficit disorder, dyslexia, or other learning disabilities (Binder & Watkins, 1990; Johnson & Layng, 1992). One of the central training centers at Morningside Academy is so confident about its success with underperforming students that it offers to reimburse parents if their child does not make 2 years' gain within 1 school year (Johnson & Street, 2004).

Support for Experience-Based Learning

General comparisons between the discrete trial format and the natural language paradigm showed that children learned and generalized better in natural learning interactions and that parents preferred this teaching format (Delprato, 2001). Children also mastered tasks faster when given natural, rather than artificial, reinforcers (Koegel, O'Dell, & Dunlap, 1988). Given the nature of autism, it makes sense that children learn concepts faster when they have previous experience with them. A child asked to differentiate opposites such as *full* and *empty* without having any experience with these concepts is less likely to learn and generalize them than a peer who has played countless times pouring water into containers or pretending to drink from empty cups. In my experience, when given a ball that does not bounce because it has little air, children quickly master requesting the "full" ball, using terms such as the "okay ball" or the "good ball" or even demanding the "nonflat ball."

Support for Visual Strategies

Until the 1980s, nonverbal children, adolescents, and adults with ASD usually were trained in communicating through *sign language* (Kiernan, 1981). When comparing the learning rates of children with Down syndrome and children with ASD, researchers found that children with ASD learned faster to discriminate pictures and to communicate through word cards, while children with Down syndrome were better at learning new imitations and communicating through hand signs (Bernard-Opitz, 1983). Pictures and word cards, therefore, should be considered as nonverbal communication tools for children with ASD. The choice of a communication system should not depend only on evidence of learning rates in discriminating shapes, letters, and word cards and in imitating hand signs. The choice also depends on the child's social environment; the attitudes of parents, teachers, and siblings may either support a system or make it futile.

Since 1985, PECS (Frost & Bondy, 1985, 2002) has become very popular and has helped many children with ASD. In one study, when vocal imitation, hand signs, and PECS were trained simultaneously, six of seven children learned PECS but failed to learn the others. Only one of the children learned to imitate sounds and hand signs (Bondy & Frost, 1994). Of 85 nonverbal preschool children with ASD, 95% learned the PECS system. In conjunction with PECS, 76% even learned to talk (Bondy & Frost, 1994).

At the Princeton Institute in Princeton, N.J., pictured activity schedules were used beginning in 1986. This method helped children with ASD predict events; understand sequences in everyday activities, such as going shopping or building with Lego blocks; and expect certain reinforcers. With the aid of pictured activity schedules, four boys ages 9 to 14 years were able to keep themselves busy in their group home for 99% of the time (MacDuff, Krantz, & McClannahan, 1993).

As mentioned previously, the TEACCH program is based on visual support and meaningful teaching targets and has become well known in many countries of the world (Mesibov, 1997). TEACCH training is offered throughout the United States, Europe, Australia, and Asia. Even though it is one of the evidence-based practices recommended for people with autism, the TEACCH program is rarely compared to other treatment methods. In one of the few investigations with 16 matched children, researchers found that TEACCH training yielded better outcomes as compared to education in an integrated classroom (Panerai, Ferrante, & Zingale, 2002). Although comparison research such as this is not very common, it is highly relevant.

SUMMARY

Since the first descriptions of autism, many different interventions have been employed in the treatment of children with autism. Behavioral, structured, and experience/activity/play-based approaches are at the forefront of methods researched and recommended for this population. This chapter provided examples and rationales for the discrete trial format, precision teaching, pivotal response training, experience/activity/play-based approaches, as well as visual methods such as PECS, TEACCH, and activity schedules. Even though there is evidence supporting these specific interventions, comparison research is rare. At this point the choice of specific teaching strategies depends on the nature of autism, the individual child, and the targeted teaching goal.

Managing Behavior Problems

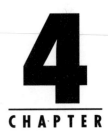

4

CHAPTER

Chapter Overview

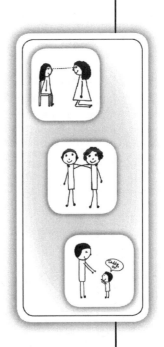

UNDERSTANDING CHALLENGING BEHAVIORS

Behavior problems or so-called "challenging" behaviors can be compared to an iceberg. Like the tip of the iceberg, behaviors such as tantrums, aggression, noncompliance, compulsions, self-injurious behavior, or echolalia can be seen clearly. However, the underlying reasons for these behaviors become evident only when one searches beneath the surface; this can be done by conducting a behavior analysis (Schopler & Mesibov, 1994). Recent evidence has indicated that a child's behavior problems serve a function, and, therefore, the problem behaviors can be reduced only if their functions are understood (Durand & Merges, 2001). Comparable to the medical model where treatment of a runny nose caused by a cold is different from that caused by an allergy, behavior problems first need to be understood in terms of their function before deciding on treatment. The main functions of behavior problems are request for attention, demand avoidance, need for stimulation, satisfaction of compulsive tendencies, and physical needs (Durand & Crimmins, 1988). Figure 4.1 shows these causes. The iceberg analogy has been used to show behavior symptoms as observable behaviors that have underlying causes (Schopler & Mesibov, 1994).

It is useful to note that many of the unusual behaviors of people with autism have functions similar to those of the behaviors of people without ASD. When typical children and adults are bored, they may engage in self-stimulatory behavior, such as wiggling their feet, rocking their chairs, twirling their hair, or biting their fingernails. To some extent, a boy who deliberately burps in class can be compared to a manager who talks continuously, just to get attention. The girl who develops a stomachache right before a class test avoids a stressful situation, as does a child with ASD who hits himself whenever given a disliked demand.

Similarly, the behaviors of typical children and adults also can be motivated by sensory feedback. We scratch a mosquito bite to reduce the itch, or rotate a foot to activate circulation. Often, however, the reasons underlying behavior problems are not so obvious in people with autism. Therefore, therapists must make systematic observations and examine questionnaire data to determine root causes of behavior. Observation will be discussed later in the chapter.

Request for Attention

A frequent function of behavior problems in children with autism is the request for attention.

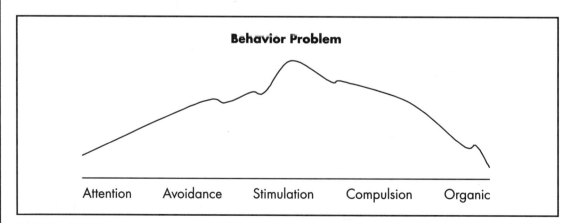

FIGURE 4.1. Main functions of behavior problems.

In class, 8-year-old Austin would hit his chin hard and continuously with his fist, causing his chin to bleed. Whenever his teacher turned to him and tried to calm him down, Austin stopped hitting himself; whenever she turned away, he went back to his self-injurious behavior.

This case shows that loving attention alone is not sufficient to reduce problems in the long run; in fact, attention actually can make problems worse. It is therefore important to understand the specific function of the problem behavior and to select a consequence that matches the function. In Austin's case the behavior was immediately reduced when we showed him that the gesture "come here" was as effective in getting the teacher's attention as the hitting behavior. This intervention, teaching Austin to communicate appropriately, is an example of differential reinforcement of communication, which means that Austin learns to express himself more appropriately through alternative means.

> **Differential reinforcement of communication is an important alternative to behavior problems.**

Demand Avoidance

The problem behaviors of some children occur predominantly under demand conditions. These behaviors are motivated by escape or avoidance and can take different forms, such as noncompliance, oppositional behavior, frequent mistakes, or even physical attacks.

Nonverbal, 13-year-old Michael attacks his teacher daily when she meets him from the school bus and tries to escort him to his table in class. As a result of the difficult passage between bus and classroom, Michael often is shoved into a beanbag chair by the hapless teacher, where he then spends the rest of the school day without further risk of demands.

In behavioral terminology, this case shows positive reinforcement of avoidance behavior. To find out what is causing Michael's attacks, his teacher could conduct a systematic analysis that would identify triggers for Michael's behavior problem. Answers to the following questions will be telling: Is Michael also aggressive when a different person picks him up from the bus, someone whom he associates with positive experiences, such as swimming or music? Is he also aggressive when he knows there will be positive settings in his class, such as his breakfast, liked toys, soothing music, or easy tasks? Such changes in daily events can reduce severe behavior problems and set the stage for positive interactions.

In the above scenario, other changes could also be adopted. Can Michael learn to indicate his wishes through pictures, word cards, or gestures ("Stop," "Break," "Pool," "No")? Would a pictured daily schedule help Michael to predict what is happening at what time and know when his beloved beanbag time, swimming session, or a break is scheduled? Could the teaching goals be made easier, more functional, and more motivating? Figure 4.2 shows an example of a picture schedule.

Sensory Stimulation

Behavior problems in children with ASD can function as sensory stimulation. Children may wave their hands or objects, spin objects or themselves, pick up and drop sand or water endlessly,

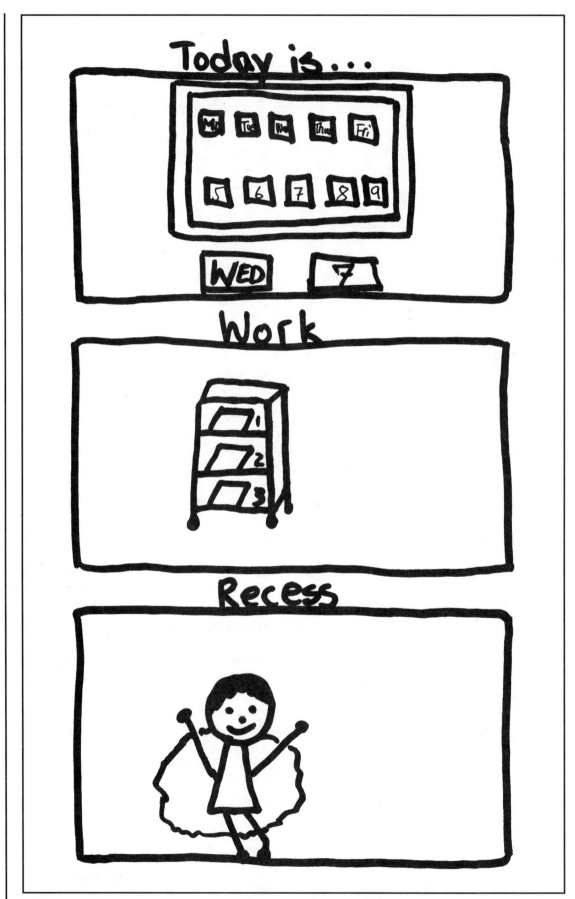

FIGURE 4.2. Picture or word sequences allow children to visualize daily events and help reduce potential behavior problems.

or make stereotypic sounds by clapping, knocking, or shaking objects. Repetitive jumping, bouncing, and other continuous rocking movements seem to be favorite activities of many children with ASD. In a classic experiment, Rincover (1978) tried to understand the reasons for one of these favorite self-stimulations: the stereotypic spinning of a plate by a boy with ASD. Rincover first blocked the view of the plate by blindfolding the boy, then later masked the sound by letting the boy spin the plate only on carpet. It was obvious that the boy was mainly interested in the sound, not the sight, of the plate. Rincover offered the boy a music box as an alternative to the plate, and the boy shifted his interest to the more appropriate play activity. This study showed that one of the first steps to understanding self-stimulation is to determine whether the behavior has visual, auditory, tactile, or vestibular components. The therapist must then pinpoint which component interests the child and search for a more appropriate alternative in the same modality.

> **Alternatives to sensory stimulation should be offered in the same modality as the self-stimulation.**

Compulsive Behaviors

Compulsive behaviors and insistence on sameness test the tolerance levels of family members, peers, and teachers. Children line up objects, touch or drop them repetitively, open and close doors and drawers, and turn lights on and off. People with ASD engage in such compulsive behavior, regardless of age, level of disability, or culture.

For a long time, a 10-year-old American girl refused to sleep without wearing her mother's high heels and her grandmother's hat. A Singaporean girl of the same age screamed for hours if her routine was interrupted. She would go to school wearing her socks, but always insisted on leaving the school without wearing them.

A German 4-year-old girl insisted on having a bowel movement only in the potty while riding in the car. Another boy refused to leave the house without taking his pet fish in a plastic bag.

A 5-year-old Singaporean boy was dismissed from kindergarten because he persisted in covering his ears, throwing a tantrum, and trying to leave the group whenever the children sang their morning songs.

Many children with ASD have tantrums and are nervous when their routines or expectations are interrupted. These can be small, simple changes, such as when the car makes an unusual turn, the teacher has a new hairstyle or glasses, the swimming lesson is canceled, a puzzle piece is missing, or the group members do not all cross their legs in the expected manner. When rituals or compulsions are not permitted, some children panic. There are endless examples of these kinds of scenarios, showing the tragic-comic side of living with people with ASD. In many cases, the indicated problems are motivated by the child's wish to structure the environment and make it more predictable.

> **Announcing changes, developing clear structures, and providing visual sequences can help reduce a child's anxiety, paving the way for learning more appropriate behavior.**

It is often difficult to understand compulsive behaviors such as unusual fascinations. Why are some children interested in drains or grids, instantly searching for them in every house they enter? Why do other children consider specific shapes, letters, or numbers fascinating? While there usually are no understandable reasons for the specific obsessions or compulsions, their use as sensory reinforcers has been helpful (Rincover, Cook, Peoples, & Packard, 1979).

More acceptable are special talents, which can be seen in about 10% of children with ASD. Some children, for example, are *hyperlexic* at the age of 2 years, having developed precocious reading skills without any specific instruction (Siegel, 2003). Others learn maps or train and bus schedules in no time, remember dates of birthdays, calculate calendar dates, have a photographic memory, and other skills. Some develop savant skills in areas as diverse as mathematical calculation, sports trivia, or music, such as being able to play an advanced piano piece after hearing it only once. Famous people with ASD have shared their personal perspective on autism and have managed to show the positive side of this other way of being. Temple Grandin, for example, has turned her skill of thinking in pictures into a highly applauded specialist skill in developing holding places for captured animals (Grandin & Scariano, 1986). Savant artists such as Gilles Trehin (2004) share their fascination with details in highly detailed paintings, showing amazing talent and unusual fantasies (Schwaab, 1992).

Biological Basis

Recent neurobiological and genetic research has clearly demonstrated a biological basis for some behavior problems, such as self-stimulation and self-injurious behavior. It has been demonstrated that self-injurious behavior can lead to elevated levels of certain neurotransmitters (Thompson et al., 1995), thereby possibly normalizing required sensory stimulation. Medications have been found that influence either neurotransmitters or the endogenous opiad system (see Symons, Thompson, & Rodriguez, 2004). Opiad antagonists, such as naltrexone have been the most effective medication in reducing self-injurious behavior in 50% to 80% of subjects (White & Schultz, 2000).

CONDUCTING A BEHAVIOR ANALYSIS

The most productive way to determine what functions problem behaviors serve is to interview parents and knowledgeable others, make systematic observations of the person with ASD, and conduct experimental analysis (Durand & Merges, 2001; Iwata et al., 1982). The following questions should be part of a behavior interview·

- What specific behavior is observed?
- How often and for how long does it occur?
- In what setting does it happen or not happen?
- Which consequences are useful?

These questions are discussed in detail next.

How To Observe Specific Behavior

To allow an objective observation by independent parties, behavior problems need to be defined in observable terms. This so-called operationalization is the basis for agreement on specific therapy goals by parents and teachers and allows for consistent handling of the problem and documentation of its change. A label for behavior such as *aggressive* or *disobedient* is not sufficient for independent observation (Baker et al., 2004). Aggression, for example, can entail destruction of material and verbal or physical abuse, or it can refer to a child's specific tendency to chase the neighbor's cat and pull its tail. Like aggression, disobedience comes in many forms. The problem behavior must be made specific. An example of a good operational definition of disobedience, or noncompliance, would be as follows: "David does not respond to an instruction within 3 seconds." As defined, this problem behavior can be more easily observed and measured.

Frequency and Duration

Before starting a diet, most people first check their current weight for a couple of days. In the same way, a baseline of the frequency or duration of the problem behavior also should be conducted before the start of any intervention. Observation periods should be consistent (such as at 10-minute intervals) and occur during times when the behavior is likely to happen. The behavior must be measured long enough to obtain a stable variation of the data, which usually takes about 1 week. While frequency counts are sufficient for many behaviors, others may need the duration (e.g., tantrums) or the intensity (e.g., physical assault) measured. Once the data show a consistent trend, therapy can start. The effect of the behavioral intervention can be monitored as data are continuously gathered.

Setting

Once a behavior is operationalized, various observers can determine whether it occurs in specific situations and with specific people. Observers can see whether a child is more compliant with the teacher or with the mother or whether the child complies better while in a play or a work situation. It also is valuable to know where or when behaviors do not occur; therefore, observation throughout the day is important. It might be found that the child who is said to wave objects continuously does not actually do so on the bus or in the bathtub.

PREVENTING AND REDUCING PROBLEM BEHAVIORS

A core finding of learning theory is that behavior is determined by preceding events, also called *antecedents,* as well as *consequences,* which follow a behavior. By changing preceding events, or triggers, behavior problems can be reduced or eliminated. Furthermore, positive consequences increase the likelihood that a behavior will be repeated, while negative ones decrease the likelihood. Consider the following example:

Antecedent	Behavior	Consequence	Likely effect
• Family is having dinner.			
• Child is passed his plate.	• Child pushes plate off table and cries.	• Mother comforts child. • Mother picks up child's plate and feeds child.	• Child's problem behavior is reinforced and likely to happen again.
		• Child has to pick up his plate and has to clean the floor.	• Child's problem behavior is punished and less likely to happen again.

Understanding the above example of trigger behavior problems and consequences is a basis for successful behavior intervention. Behavior problems can be prevented through various means, changing either setting events, the physical or social environment, or consequences. Many problems can be eliminated through environmental changes. A child who rocks his chair may stop if the chair is placed against the wall. For another child, the presence of her mother during her first therapy sessions may prevent tantrums and lack of attention to the task. Antecedents can be physical or psychological factors, such as pain, hunger, thirst, fatigue, or toilet needs, or sensory problems, like an itchy T-shirt label. Other triggers can be found in the social setting or the specific task demand. If attention-getting functions maintain the problem behavior, it is useful to ignore it and to develop appropriate alternatives. Figure 4.3 illustrates the relationship between antecedents, behavior problems, and consequences.

Developing Alternative Behaviors

A child spent his time juggling stones and other nonedibles, which he often swallowed. This high-risk behavior was replaced by more appropriate play, juggling balls.

The above strategy, called differential reinforcement of other behavior (DRO), is often used when the problem behavior serves self-stimulatory purposes. Self-stimulation can also be reduced by differential reinforcement of incompatible behavior (DRI), which means that some behaviors cannot physically be performed when doing others. For example, children who spin or wave objects tend not to do so when riding a bike, skiing, swimming, or carrying something in both hands. Because many behaviors are communicative, the development of communicative alternatives, or differential reinforcement of communicative behavior (DRC), is another important intervention. In this method, the communicative intent of a behavior problem is analyzed, and the therapist develops a more appropriate verbal or nonverbal communication to serve the same function as the behavior problem.

In the workshop, 18-year-old Todd would get very upset when the person next to him would take his screws without asking. Todd learned to pass a card saying, "Ask please" to the other person, which resulted in a kinder interaction for both parties.

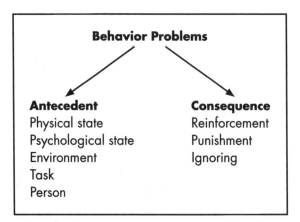

FIGURE 4.3. The ABC's of behavior analysis: antecedent, behavior, and consequence.

Other Methods for Reducing Behavior Problems

Punishment refers to aversive consequences that lead to a reduction of the problem behavior. Punishment can take two forms: withdrawal of a positive consequence or the addition of an aversive contingency. A child who bites his nails, rocks, fights with his siblings, or scatters popcorn while watching TV will soon learn that these behaviors are not appreciated if the parents turn off the TV every time these behaviors occur. This withdrawal of a positive consequence is a form of time-out. The child could also be asked to leave the TV room or sit on a time-out chair for a short period of time. Other aversive consequences, such as physically restraining the child or making him pick up the popcorn and clean the entire living-room floor (called overcorrection), may also reduce the behavior. Because physical restraint and overcorrection are more restrictive than turning off the TV, ethical issues need to be considered. Behavior intervention should always be based on the least restrictive and most effective alternative. Figure 4.4 shows a hierarchy of methods to reduce behavior problems, ranging from preventive methods, such as changing the environment, to more aversive methods, such as time-out. The hierarchy should be read from bottom to top, left to right.

In developing useful consequences, that is, consequences that serve to reduce the problem behavior, parents and teachers should consider the individual child. A positive consequence for one child may be a negative consequence for another. A child with ASD may perceive a well-intended hug or kiss as aversive, and there are even some children with autism who like to be scolded. The decision about whether a behavior leads to a positive or a negative consequence is best made by looking at the specific likes and dislikes of the child.

Punishing in the strict sense of the word
Time-out
Physical restraint
Overcorrection

Removing the positives
Interruption of a liked situation or activity
Time-out from a liked object
Time-out from a liked person
Reduction of privileges

Ignoring and reinforcing alternative behavior
Differential reinforcement of other behavior
Differential reinforcement of incompatible behavior
Differential reinforcement of communication

Preventing the problem
Change the environment
Distraction

FIGURE 4.4. Hierarchy of methods to reduce behavior problems.

SUMMARY

It is important to note that every problem behavior serves a certain function for the child. Through a functional behavior analysis, antecedents and reinforcing or punishing consequences can be assessed. The main functions problem behaviors serve are a request for attention, avoidance or escape of demands, self-stimulation and compulsion, and handling organic needs. The specific intervention chosen must serve the same function as the problem behavior for the intervention to be effective. Frequency, duration, or intensity of the problem should be monitored prior to and during the intervention to make sure it is reducing the unwanted behavior.

Reinforcing Behavior

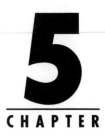

Chapter Overview

What Reinforcers Are Available?

What Are Token Systems?

How Does One Find the Most Effective Reinforcement?

Summary

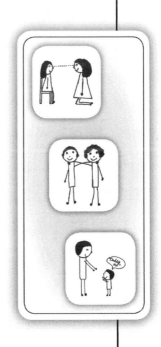

any parents, teachers, and therapists of children with ASD hope that praise and acknowledgement are sufficient to reinforce appropriate behavior. There generally is no
doubt that typically developing children benefit from praise and grades as incentive for
learning, but such symbolic reinforcers do not work for most children with ASD. Well-meaning
parents and teachers often reject material or activity reinforcement because of their similarity to
"teaching dogs a trick." Unfortunately, this attitude often creates an additional hurdle for many
children with ASD. In the beginning of therapy many autistic children do not understand that
positive consequences follow hard efforts. To overcome motivation problems, lack of social perception, and language barriers, such reinforcing consequences are highly necessary. Parents and
teachers must overcome their prejudices to give children with ASD a chance to reach long-term
goals such as self-motivated learning, understanding of subtle social reinforcement, and—last
but not least—a regular paid job (which seems quite close to material reinforcement).

WHAT REINFORCERS ARE AVAILABLE?

Quite simply, positive reinforcers are consequences liked by the child that increase the likelihood of a particular behavior's occurring again. In the beginning of teaching a child with
problems understanding contingencies, material reinforcers such as getting access to liked toys,
sensory stimulation, or food serve as a good starting point. In later stages of therapy, praise, high
fives, and so forth should be sufficient. Positive reinforcers can be divided into four categories:
social, symbolic, activity, and material. Figure 5.1 shows the hierarchy of positive reinforcers
and should be read from left to right.

Consequences that directly follow desired behavior, such as receiving verbal praise or
getting a hug, are called *immediate reinforcers*. *Delayed reinforcers*, on the other hand, follow a
time lapse, such as receiving grades at the end of a school term or pay at the end of the month.

Material
Self-stimulation
Toys
Food, drinks

Activity
Outings to the park, city, or zoo
Swinging, swimming
TV, computer games

Symbolic
Tokens
Grades
Privileges, roles

Social
Praise, acknowledgement
Physical contact, closeness
Interaction, games

FIGURE 5. 1. Hierarchy of positive reinforcers to develop behavior.

Reinforcers can also be distinguished as *positive* or *negative*, both following a behavior and increasing its chance to occur again. Negative reinforcers are like a tight shoe or demanding homework. If you avoid the pain by taking the shoe off or ignoring the difficult homework, the immediate consequence is relief, which is reinforcing. Escape and avoidance behavior may have negative repercussions in the long run, at least in the example of the ignored homework. On the other hand, they can be powerful incentives for children with ASD, who often learn fast to shake their head, make a "no" gesture, or show the "Break" word card to reject or terminate an activity.

Research by Koegel and his colleagues has indicated that consequences related to the behavior are more effective than consequences that are unrelated to the behavior. In the past, therapists tended to reinforce a child for saying "ball" with a completely unrelated reinforcer, such as a piece of candy. Today, therapists know that functional consequences are more effective than artificial ones, such as allowing the child to play with the ball after she says "ball" (R. Koegel & Williams, 1980).

Children are more motivated when task demands make sense and when the scope of a task, such as the number of items one has to complete, is obvious. A study by R. Koegel and Williams (1980) demonstrated that autistic children had increased enthusiasm when they were expected to take many cloth pegs off the rim of a box, rather than taking only one off repetitively with the therapist undoing (i.e., putting the peg back on the rim) what the child had just done (i.e., taking it off). Children learn rapidly when asked to open bags or boxes, even managing difficult fine-motor or problem-solving activities, such as getting scissors to cut strings and open packages, to get access to liked items.

The sorting box shown in Figure 5.2 is another example of reinforcement embedded directly in the task (R. Koegel & Williams, 1980). A child inserts shapes into matching holes in the box. Once the child has mastered sorting the shapes, he is allowed to press the middle button to activate the box's spinning motion. The simple principle behind this method is sometimes called "Grandma's rule," meaning that "you first do what you have to do before you do what you like to do."

In therapy and in everyday settings, children often are not aware of the number of tasks or chores they have to do. And parents and therapists tend to push for more tasks once a child has successfully completed a demand. Some children notice this vicious cycle of having to work

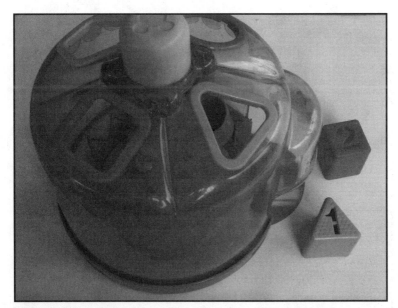

FIGURE 5. 2. In this reinforcing activity, the child places all the shapes in the correct slots, then is allowed to press the middle button to activate the spinning mechanism of the shape sorter.

more after doing well and resort to working especially slowly, making many mistakes or showing complete task avoidance. Here, the TEACCH approach discussed in previous chapters makes a lot of sense, exposing children to a predictable number of tasks that are placed in a "finish box" upon completion. Mastery and completion are powerful reinforcers for many children with ASD (Schopler et al., 2004). The setup in Figure 5.3 shows children the number of tasks they need to do.

In addition, many studies have shown that variable reinforcers and reinforcers chosen by the child lead to increased learning compared to fixed reinforcers determined by the therapist (Dunlap & Koegel, 1980; Van Houten & Nau, 1980).

What makes tasks and reinforcers most effective?

- The child should consider the tasks useful.
- Reinforcers should be matched to the individual child's interests and current needs.
- Reinforcers should have a functional relation to the task.
- Reinforcers should change from task to task and day to day.
- The child and his or her parents should decide what could serve as reinforcement.
- The task structure should indicate how much and what the child has to do.

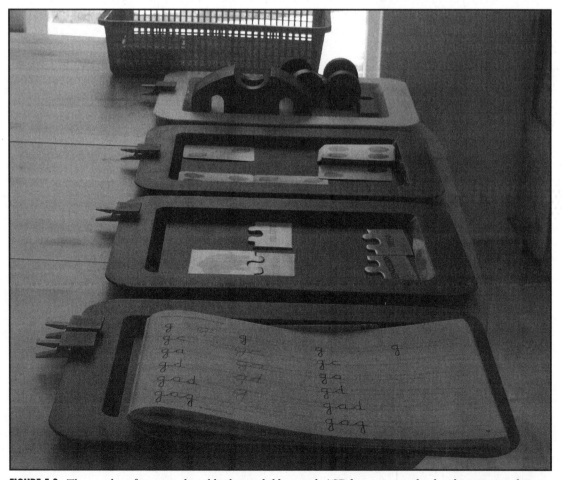

FIGURE 5.3. The number of trays on the table shows children with ASD how many tasks they have to complete.

WHAT ARE TOKEN SYSTEMS?

Tokens are symbolic reinforcers that a child receives for completing a task. They are tangible proof that reinforcement is on the way, thereby bridging the gap from immediate reinforcement to higher level delayed reinforcement. Tokens can take many forms, such as checkers, plastic chips, small cloth pegs, puzzle pieces, paper clips, beads, blocks, stickers, or even real coins. For example, the therapist can attach Velcro to the backs of the tokens, then set up a row of matching Velcro on a piece of paper or a ruler. The child can place a token on one of the Velcro pieces and see how many tokens it will take to receive the preferred item. To use tokens effectively, the therapist sets up a visual token system that shows children how many tokens are needed to obtain a preferred item. Beads can be placed on stands and pegs or puzzle pieces can be inserted into trays so that the number of necessary tokens is clear by the length of the bead stand or the number of slots in a tray.

To familiarize the child with a token economy, the therapist gives the child a small reinforcer for one token given for an easy behavior. Even responding to a simple command such as "Sit down" can be sufficient to receive a reinforcer. During the following trials, the number of tokens necessary to receive the reinforcer is increased.

The following box lists the parts of token systems.

Components of Token Systems

- List of the child's likes, interests, and reinforcers
- Cost of the reinforcers
- Hierarchy of liked items
- List of tasks and demands
- Cost of tasks

In Figure 5.4, a picture of the selected reinforcer, a ball in this case, is placed on the top area of the tray. The lower Velcro pieces indicate that the child needs three tokens to receive the indicated reinforcer.

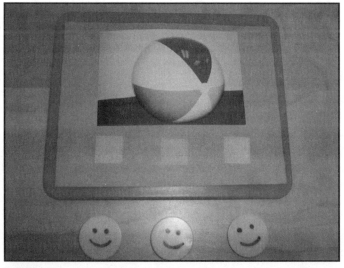

FIGURE 5.4. In this token system, the child must earn three tokens to receive the pictured ball.

For some children, a picture of a reinforcer can be cut into several pieces. In the example shown in Figure 5.5, the child receives the ice cream cone for completing the first task component, followed by one or more scoops and a topping for successive trials. Each piece equals one token, and once the child has all the pieces, he or she receives the reinforcer.

In general, therapists gradually decrease the external reinforcement system over the course of the therapy sessions, so that children learn to work for internal reinforcement and delay external gratification. After some time in a token economy, children can work one whole week to participate in a special outing during the weekend. If possible, children should participate in the development of a token system and should be involved in deciding whether they want to work for less-attractive items, which require fewer tokens and effort, or more-attractive items, which require long-term effort. A long-term goal is the development of self-efficacy, which makes children confident about taking up new challenges (Schopler et al., 2004).

How Does One Find the Most Effective Reinforcement?

The following lists summarize the use of reinforcers.

How does one find reinforcers?
- Observation
- Interviews with involved others
- Interviews with the child

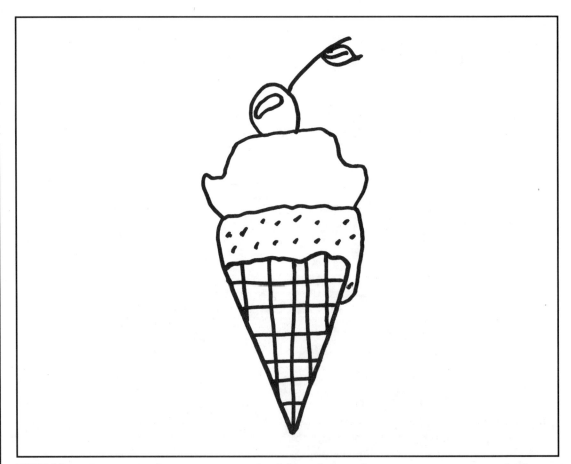

FIGURE 5.5. In this example of an ice cream cone, the child needs four tokens to get an ice cream: one for the cone, two for two scoops, and one for the cherry.

What features should reinforcers have?

- Not freely available
- Attractive
- Variable

How should the reinforcers be used?

- At first, immediately and continuously
- Later, on an intermittent basis
- Paired with praise
- Paired with comments

The parents of 14-year-old Tim were very depressed and said that they and their son's teacher had given up trying to influence their son's behavior. The boy's main activity consisted of pacing up and down waving a string. It was obvious that the string could become a reinforcer for more appropriate behavior. Fortunately I had some string in our clinic and cut a piece, allowing the boy to play with it for 10 seconds. I then took it away and asked him to sit down. Because he did not re-act, we used a slight physical prompt to get the sitting behavior. Again Tim was allowed to play with the string for 10 seconds. Once he understood the contingency between his behavior and the string, other skills could be developed, such as completing various puzzles, matching tasks, and imitation and language tasks. Because the string-waving attracted a lot of attention, I devised a way to make it easier for the parents to face the crowds of students on campus when leaving the therapy appointments. I cut Tim's string into small pieces at the end of the therapy. He lost his interest in the string because it no longer was useful for waving. He threw it away and his parents could leave the clinic without a lot of attention.

Nonverbal, 3-year-old Marcel had not learned that positive behavior leads to positive consequences. Whenever his requests were not immediately answered, he would tantrum and throw himself on the floor. Because his behavior was highly disturbing, no childcare center would accept him. His mother revealed that one of Marcel's favorite activities was to watch a certain videotape again and again. I rescheduled the therapy session for the following week, requesting that the mother bring the videotape. My first target was to get the boy to comply with the simple command to sit down in front of the TV. Marcel quickly understood that brief episodes of his favorite tape were contingent on his behavior. I managed to use this incentive to teach the imitation of knocking on the table, throwing beads in a tin can, and inserting puzzle pieces. His mother was very pleased with these first experiences of positive behavior control.

For many parents and teachers, the use of motivating consequences is often a first step to success. Many parents and teachers come to use reinforcers out of frustration because their children or students have failed to learn. The reinforcers mentioned in this chapter should only be considered as stepping stones on the way to the child's perceiving the therapist or parent as an important reinforcer who is helpful, supportive, and fun throughout the interactions. The sole use of self-stimulations or special interests as reinforcers is not recommended.

To choose potential reinforcers, parents and therapists should observe the child and determine his or her interests. The child may be attracted to various objects with sensory effects, for example (see Figure 5.6). In addition, parents, teachers, and others familiar with the autistic child can fill out a checklist of potential reinforcers (see Appendix 5.A).

For children with a good level of language comprehension, consequences should be explained and visualized as described below. Verbal or written announcements of positive or negative consequences to certain behaviors tend to be useful because being able to predict consequences helps children develop positive behaviors that will lead to positive consequences (Flick, 1998).

Examples for verbal or written announcement of consequences

If you	then
• brush your teeth without reminder	I will read you a story
• do not interrupt	you can go for a swing
• clean your room	you can watch TV
• finish your homework	you can ride your bike

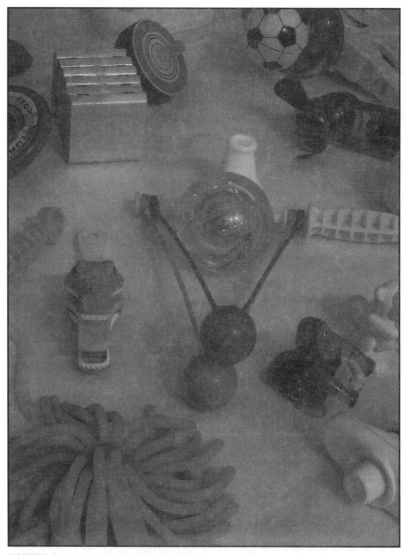

FIGURE 5.6a. Examples of visual reinforcers.

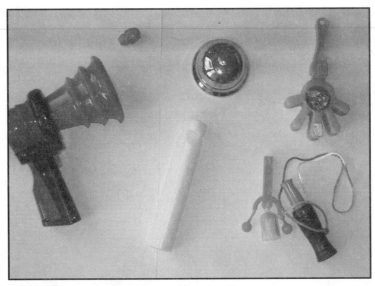

FIGURE 5.6b. Examples of auditory reinforcers.

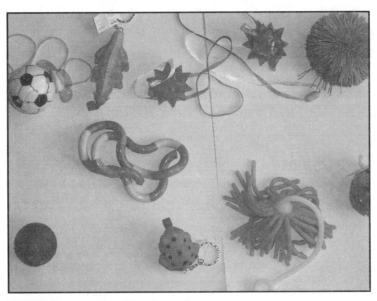

FIGURE 5.6c. Examples of tactile reinforcers.

SUMMARY

The development of appropriate behavior depends, to a large extent, on the choice of an effective reinforcer. Effective consequences can be determined by observing the child and interviewing knowledgeable others. Therapists should explore several types of reinforcers, such as material reinforcers like sensory toys, symbolic reinforcers like tokens, and social reinforcers, like praise and rough play. If at all possible, reinforcers should be natural and functional. The final goal is that the therapist and parent become the main reinforcer by being associated with positive experiences, be it reinforcing activities or objects, manageable tasks, or fun interactions. For some children, the goal may even go beyond this by making them confident and proud to master any changes.

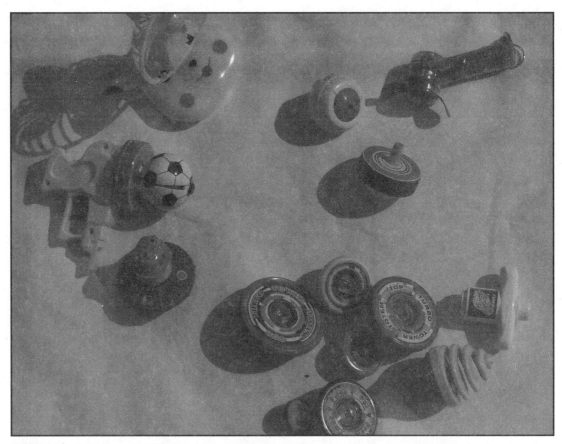

FIGURE 5.6d. Children with ASD often like spinning objects. These can be used as reinforcers.

List of Potential Reinforcers

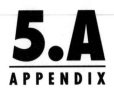

5.A

APPENDIX

Type of Stimulus	Specific Details About Stimulus	Likes	Neutral	Dislikes	Comments
Social					
Praise					
Hugs					
Strokes					
Kisses					
Tickling					
Rough play					
Songs					
Other					
Food					
Sweets					
Salty					
Sour					
Drinks					
Other					
Toys					
Puzzles					
Cars					
Trains					
Dolls					

© 2007 by PRO-ED, Inc.

Type of Stimulus	Specific Details About Stimulus	Likes	Neutral	Dislikes	Comments
Toys (cont.)					
Balls					
Cause–effect toys					
Construction toys					
Fantasy games					
Other					
Sensory Toys					
Bubbles					
Balloons					
Foam					
Water					
Sand					
Spinning objects					
Sound makers					
Musical instruments					
Vibrating objects					
Tactile objects					
Other					
Action Reinforcers					
Trampoline					

© 2007 by PRO-ED, Inc.

Type of Stimulus	Specific Details About Stimulus	Likes	Neutral	Dislikes	Comments
Action Reinforcers (*cont*)					
Gymnastics ball					
Swing					
Slide					
See-saw					
Bicycle or tricycle					
Rollerblades or ice skates					
Swimming					
Computer					
TV or videotape					
Electronic games					
Other					
Heightened Interests					
Numbers					
Letters					
Reading					
Colors or shapes					
Other					

© 2007 by PRO-ED, Inc.

Preparing for Therapy

Chapter Overview

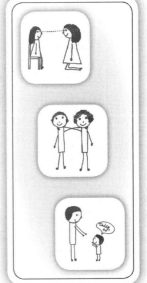

This chapter describes some of the conditions therapists must consider before therapy with a child begins in earnest, including setting up the teaching environment, conducting the first session, choosing either child-centered or therapist-centered procedures, presenting materials, using pictures, and developing a therapy plan.

Setting Up the Teaching Environment

The location of the therapy, the setup, the seating position, and the presentation of material can vary based on the age of the child, his or her personality, and the specific therapy goals. For a young, severely involved child, a table-task setting with repeated trials may be more useful than the less predictable and more varied play-type teaching environment. For a more advanced child, natural teaching situations in his or her room, the playground, or the kindergarten can be structured in such a way as to elicit the target behavior. The setting of the young, severely involved child illustrates the discrete trial format, which usually requires mass trials conducted in a table-type setting. The scenario for the more advanced child exemplifies experience-based teaching, which can be done in everyday settings.

Precision teaching and the TEACCH program tend to be conducted in table-task settings, but also can be carried out effectively in natural environments. Examples of such tasks include giving change to a cashier or crossing the street. Precision teaching, with its repetitive trials conducted in brief time intervals, requires undisturbed practice in table-task settings with generalization to natural settings as a major objective. Sorting, imitation, and preacademic and academic exercises may be easier to teach in more controlled environments, whereas most play, social, and self-help skills should be taught in natural settings.

Discrete Trial Format

Usually discrete trial format sessions are conducted in distraction-free environments with the child sitting at a table facing the therapist. The teaching target is determined before the session by the therapeutic team, and this method features simple instructions, effective prompts, and reinforcing consequences. Often material such as everyday objects, colors, shapes, or picture cards are presented in small trays, boxes, or baskets to allow for a fast succession of tasks. The response of the child is recorded as *correct, prompted,* or *incorrect*. Tokens and various individual reinforcers should be available, such as those pictured in Figure 6.1.

Precision Teaching

Precision teaching is conducted in table-task settings and in natural environments. Children may work on labeling objects as fast as they can, finding as many alternatives to overused expressions, so-called "dead" words, such as *to say* or *to get* or coming up with several ways to initiate play with a peer. Alternatives for replacing the word *say,* for example, include *talk, tell, question, indicate, reply, answer, demand, whisper, shout,* and *scream.* Characteristic features of precision teaching sessions are timers and standard celeration charts. The child's performance, such as the number of pictures or word cards labeled, patterns rebuilt, or imitations made, is measured in small units of 10, 20, or 60 seconds. If possible, the child monitors her or his own behavior, including setting the timer, charting performance, and reinforcing her or his own behavior once the fluency criteria have been reached.

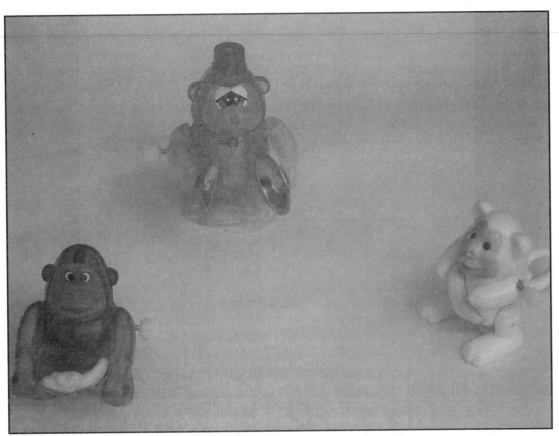

FIGURE 6.1. Positive reinforcers, such as the toys pictured, motivate children with ASD.

Experience-Based Teaching

Experience-based and natural teaching usually take place in everyday settings, be they a play setting on the floor of the child's room, the kitchen counter, or the playground. Material related to the teaching target is offered often, and the child is regularly interrupted by the teacher or caregiver, who teaches goals related to the child's experience. For example, the child who grabs a glass as a sign that she wants a drink may be stopped immediately and taught more appropriate behavior, such as how to request for the refrigerator door to be opened (e.g., saying or showing the sign or picture for "open"), to be allowed to take out a bottle of juice (e.g., "juice, please," "want juice"), and to pour the juice into the glass ("in," "juice in").

Visual Systems

Visual tasks can be done in table-type settings and natural environments. In the TEACCH program, task material is presented from left to right, corresponding to the reading direction. With this method, young children learn to match objects, pictures, or words that are the same or distinguish between those that are different. Through a similar task setup, adolescents may learn, for example, how to find the right type of battery for different flashlights or how to fill a bird feeder (Eckenrode, Fennell, & Hearsay, 2003, 2004).

To show a child how many teaching goals and tasks he will be required to do, the teacher presents a pictured or written task sequence. Photos or schematic drawings indicate what the child can expect during the day (e.g., song circle, reading, therapy session, recess, math, PE). If an activity is cancelled, its picture or card can be removed, thereby warning the child. If an activity is rescheduled, it can be moved to the anticipated new time slot. Through activity schedules, the child can be taught to complete pictured task sequences independently. If necessary, the pictured sequence can also indicate the reinforcers that follow the task completion. An example of an activity schedule is provided in Figure 6.2.

Autistic children as young as 2 years can learn to follow activity schedules to complete a series of tasks set up on trays in open shelves (see Figure 6.3). They are able to complete simple tasks, such as doing puzzles, sorting, or drawing without any assistance. The completed tasks are put into a "finish box," and the children move on to the next part of their schedules.

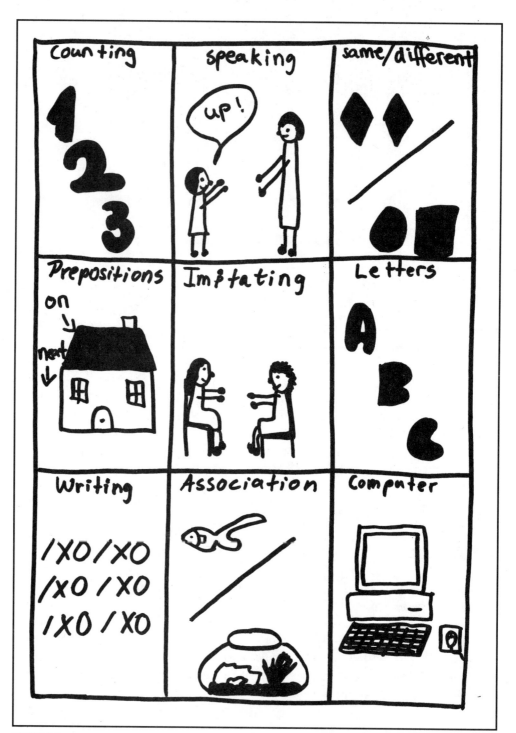

FIGURE 6.2. Pictured activity schedules show children what activities to expect.

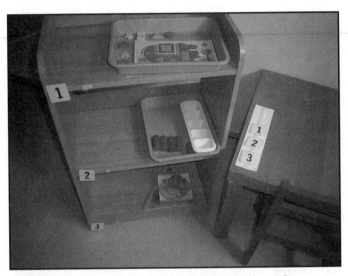

FIGURE 6.3. Children learn to follow sequences with numbers or pictures and to complete the tasks on the shelf independently (Source: Autistic Association Singapore).

CONDUCTING THE FIRST THERAPY SESSION

The first therapy sessions involving young children with ASD are often a challenge. Children may refuse to comply with any instructions, whisk material off the table, run aimlessly around the room, or tantrum, throwing themselves onto the floor. Therapists from different schools of thought may deal with all these behaviors in very different ways. The child's age, personality, level of functioning, and motivation, as well as features of the family, should be considered when making decisions about therapy approaches. In the case of severe behavior problems, trained and experienced behavior therapists must perform a functional behavior analysis. Naive therapists can cause more harm than good—even in the first session. Remember that treatment methods need to be as effective and unrestrictive as possible.

During the first contacts with a family, my colleagues and I usually ask the parents to show us, for 15 minutes, how they work or play with their child. Every 5 minutes they are asked to demonstrate a new teaching goal, such as sorting, imitating, or eliciting verbal or nonverbal communication. This introductory period makes it less likely that artificial problems will occur during the session as a result of the child's unfamiliarity with the setting or the therapist. It also gives a first impression of the parents' teaching methods and interaction with the child and of the child's general level of functioning. Video documentation can serve as a baseline against which future progress can be compared.

Selecting the right teaching environment includes making decisions on seating arrangement. In the early stages of therapy, the teacher may need to limit the child's movements to make running away less likely. This can be accomplished by using a chair with armrests or by placing the child in such a way that escape is prevented through the position of the therapist or furniture. For managing a small group of more compliant children, a teacher may find a U-shaped table useful. In general, tasks should be made so attractive that escape is the last thing on a child's mind. With improved compliance and cooperation from children, the teacher can expect that most preschoolers with ASD will work for 20 to 30 minutes on three to four tasks. Some beginning compliance or imitation tasks are easier to practice if the therapist faces the child without a table in between.

DISTINGUISHING BETWEEN CHILD-CENTERED AND THERAPIST-CENTERED PROCEDURES

In experience-based and natural language strategies, the child's initiative directs therapy, whereas in discrete trial approaches and precision teaching, the therapist drives the sessions.

For child-centered therapy approaches, the child's focus of interest starts a teaching interaction. Sensory toys or other interesting objects are placed in playpens, in play corners, or on the table to entice the child into a learning situation. Young children with high anxiety often feel safer when allowed to sit on a parent's lap or at least stay close to them.

On the other hand, therapists who use the discrete trial format or precision teaching frequently start therapy by trying to get the child to comply with simple commands, such as, "Sit down," "Come here," or "Put it in." Physical prompts often follow these first instructions so the child understands that correct responses lead to liked consequences. In other words, it pays to be good. To develop an appropriate work attitude, the therapist must conduct repetitive trials over many sessions.

As mentioned before, experienced behavior therapists must handle cases of severe behavior problems. It may be necessary to briefly hold or physically guide some children to interrupt dangerous, aggressive, or destructive behavior. Though necessary, these interventions must be carefully planned and monitored and should be discussed with all involved. Such action should be conducted with controlled emotion, such as a calm voice, as it will inevitably restrict the child's freedom. Often a breakthrough occurs when a child understands that positive behavior leads to positive reinforcement, resulting in a dramatic improvement in behavior. Within the TEACCH setting, therapists try to prevent behavior problems by engaging children in tasks and redirecting them to constructive activities.

PRESENTING MATERIALS AND USING PICTURES

The presentation of material should be as clear and as simple as possible. To allow for a smooth transition from one task to another, the therapist can organize task material into separate containers. To help children with fine-motor problems grasp and manipulate small objects such as pictures, coins, or plastic beads, the therapist can present them on a carpet square instead of the smooth surface of a table. Styrofoam trays with cutouts for rebuilding block patterns can be helpful for young children or children with more disabilities because the cutout slots indicate how many blocks are needed and where they should be placed (Payne, 2003).

All too often, the pictures used in materials are too abstract or unrelated to the experiences of children with severe disabilities. The choice of pictures should not be guided by the therapist's or the parents' idea about what is cute. Neither should it be affected by therapy materials companies that favor certain picture systems. Instead, clarity, simplicity, and functionality should be the guiding principles for picture choices. For children who cannot yet discriminate pictures, a helpful first step into picture recognition is to use photos of their favorite objects and pictures of reinforcers and the actual corresponding items.

Many children have rapidly learned to discriminate pictures in tasks where liked and disliked items are used. Imagine two objects—an attractive candy and a not-so-attractive tube of toothpaste—hidden in two boxes, in drawers, or behind specially designed flaps. Attached to the top of each box, drawer, or flap is a pictured representation of the hidden object behind it. If a boy were to choose the container with the candy picture, he would get to eat the candy. If he were to choose the toothpaste, he would get that instead, thus inspiring him to make a better choice next time. Figure 6.4 shows a divided container being used to aid in discrimination tasks.

I once visited an adolescent with severe disabilities during her breakfast time. She was nonverbal, and when I was there, she happily scooped up her cornflakes and ate them. When she tapped her spoon on the table to get some more, I showed her the box of cornflakes (with a good picture on the front) and a nearby packet of mashed potatoes. Even when the two items were placed in different locations, she would look at the box with the cornflakes picture. Whenever she looked at the box of cornflakes, I responded by pouring just a few flakes into her bowl to keep her interested, and to check that she really understood the different pictures.

Children with ASD often know that packages indicate various attractive items. Is the child able to discriminate a packet of raisins from a packet of paper clips, or a packet of cotton candy from a packet of cotton wool? My colleagues and I have witnessed astonishing discriminations with food or drink items, even in children whose teachers had indicated a lack of any discriminatory skills during regular sorting and matching tasks. Children chose Nutella or peanut butter on bread over similar-looking but less-liked spreads such as hummus or liver sausage. Similarly, we observed good color discrimination instantly when children consistently selected small cups of milk instead of less-liked coffee, tomato juice, or root beer in similar cups.

When the child is working on matching pictures and using them for communication, the therapist should find out what kinds of pictures best suit the child and consider a variety of

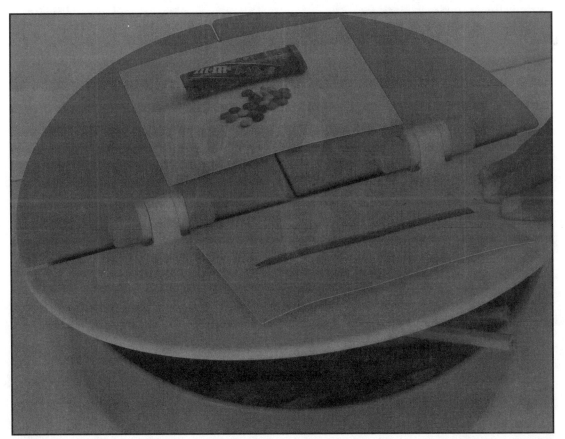

FIGURE 6.4. This task setup requires the child to pay close attention to the picture to get the liked, rather than a disliked, item.

ways in which to present them. Test to see if the child responds better to color or black-and-white photos or schematic or line drawings. Instead of responding to the common presentation of pictures on a table, some children are more motivated by taking pictures off hooks, reading stands, magnetic boards, or Velcro. Even taking them off a laundry line can be interesting. Children with advanced picture skills can be motivated by using digital photos to report on recent events.

A 7-year-old boy with ASD flew into Singapore all the way from neighboring Malaysia for his therapy. With the help of photos on his digital camera, he described the events prior to therapy, such as being at the airport in Johor Baru, flying on the plane, having breakfast, and so forth.

DEVELOPING AN INDIVIDUAL THERAPY PLAN

The development of an individual therapy plan for a child with ASD can be compared to the search for the key to open a specific lock. Just as only one key will fit the lock of a particular house, so too the specific features of a student have to be considered when devising his or her particular therapy plan. There is no undifferentiated, one-size-fits-all therapy approach for children with ASD. This is true for methods to reduce behavior problems as well as for methods to develop new skills.

A child with autism is a complex individual whose disturbances in perceiving, thinking, learning, communicating, playing, and behaving in social contexts must be considered. His or her developmental level, motivation, and interests, as well as possible secondary problems such as an attention-deficit, hyperactivity, or sleep disorder, should be included in a therapy plan. Before deciding on specific procedures, those involved with the child must discuss therapy targets and the social context.

SUMMARY

Therapy procedures can be divided into therapist-centered and child-centered methods. Established procedures for children with ASD vary in the specific location of therapy, the seating arrangements, and the presentation of material. While the discrete trial format is usually conducted at a table, precision teaching, TEACCH methods, and experience-based teaching are less restricted to a certain location but usually include everyday settings. For the success of therapy, it is important that interventions match the specific teaching targets, the individual features of the child, and his or her social context.

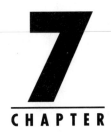

Chapter Overview

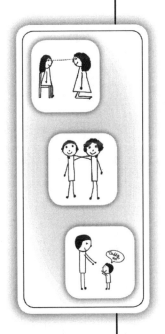

The curriculum in this chapter presents tasks aimed at developing necessary skills in children with ASD. These children often have to be taught to be attentive, to look at people, to imitate, to develop concepts, to comprehend language, to communicate in an appropriate manner, to play, and to develop independence. To match the children's learning needs with proven therapy methods, my colleagues and I developed the STEP curriculum, which combines structured teaching with experience-based and visual programs. For each therapy area four core therapy methods are demonstrated:

- Discrete trial format
- Precision teaching
- Natural and experience-based methods
- Visual systems

Parents, teachers, and therapists need to be aware that these four teaching methods should not be considered as rigid, separate approaches. Instead, they constitute a continuum of methods that are effective in teaching children with ASD. As such, these four therapy methods can be used in isolation or combined.

Because the specific training sequences for each target area follow the development of typically developing children, therapists will need to make adaptations for the characteristics of children with ASD. For these children, learning styles, communication problems, motivation issues, and individual interests have to be considered when planning treatment programs. Children with ASD, for example, have a much more difficult time using a pointing gesture to alert people to interesting objects or events as compared to typical children. Instead, they learn to point faster when pointing is used to request attractive objects or events. In general, the training sequence must be flexible enough to take into account the problems of individual children, their interests, and their motivation.

At the beginning of each of the eight curriculum areas, the relevance of the specific training unit is described. Key strategies are presented, aimed at matching the teaching method and the level of difficulty to the individual learning characteristics of the child. Reproducible forms for each area are provided in the appendix at the end of this chapter.

An overview of the STEP training sequence is presented for each curriculum area and can be used as a guideline for assessing the child's skill level and also as a general before-and-after checklist to document the effect of the intervention. Examples are given for two to four tasks per teaching method. These tasks are indicated in the sample forms provided for the training methods. Please note that these examples do not represent the wide scope of specific instructional methods and available teaching tasks. They need to be considered as flexible models for additional task descriptions, which can be developed by parents, therapists, and teachers.

The following sections offer an overview of the STEP curriculum. Readers are encouraged to collaborate with experienced professionals and to use the recommended readings for refining individual educational programs. As parents and therapists employ this curriculum, my colleagues and I hope that children with ASD will learn to reach their potential and—at the same time—have enjoyable interactions with those who teach them.

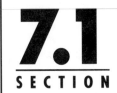
Section Overview

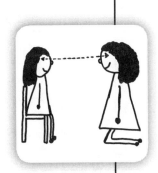

This first curriculum section focuses on the reasons for teaching attention, eye contact, and joint attention and matches specific intervention methods to features of children. The four STEP methods described earlier are exemplified with sequenced curriculum tasks.

IMPORTANCE OF ATTENTION, EYE CONTACT, AND JOINT ATTENTION

Typical infants come into the world with an inherent interest in looking at faces and a preprogrammed ability to perceive motion. The need to establish eye contact is likely biological because it plays a role in human survival. For example, throughout the generations, children have looked to the faces of their mothers to discern dangers in their environment. Eye contact enables us to share the knowledge of others and helps children in particular to evaluate the things they experience, including potentially dangerous things such as strangers, dogs, and cars.

Children with ASD, on the other hand, have notable problems attending to people, looking at faces, and engaging in joint attention (Kasari, Sigman, & Yirmiya, 1993). Many autistic children look at their interaction partners only briefly, if at all. They do not share interests and feelings with their interaction partners and fail to communicate spontaneously (Stone et al., 1997). Research has consistently demonstrated the importance of joint attention, both for early diagnosis and as a target during intervention. According to Mundy and Crowson (1997), 80% to 90% of young children diagnosed with autism can be discriminated from young children with other developmental delays because of the lack of joint attention skills in the children with autism.

What is joint attention?

Joint attention is the ability to share the experience of looking at an object or an event with another person.

Why are attention, eye contact, and joint attention important?

- Listening and looking
- Visual engagement with the conversation partner
- Visual engagement with the conversation object
- Prerequisite for learning
- Predictor of autistic disorder
- Precursor of the theory of mind (i.e., the ability to understand that others have beliefs, desires, and intentions that are different from one's own)
- Component of social behavior
- Component of communication behavior

As early as the 1970s, Gallagher and Prutting had observed that children express a wide array of communicative functions through nonverbal behavior such as eye contact, mimicry, gesturing, and posture (Gallagher & Prutting, 1983). If one follows the gaze of another person, one can often deduce his or her wishes and intentions. For instance, a glance at the sugar bowl on the breakfast table says that sugar is desired; a quick look at the clock indicates an intention to leave. In typical interactions, drawn-out eye contact can signal adoration, but it may also turn into an unpleasant stare. Joint attention is part of more advanced communication, such as requesting, questioning, and expressing likes and dislikes. Joint attention also is a direct precursor to the theory of mind.

In teaching children with ASD, proponents of discrete trial learning use the repeated request to "Look" at the partner for eye contact training, whereas those who follow developmental and linguistic models embed eye contact training in a social context (Quill, 2002). The training sequence presented here stresses early communicative functions in eye contact through the range of STEP teaching methods.

On the playground, 4-year-old Alvin repeatedly collided with other children. He ran aimlessly without consideration of those around him. In contrast, his peers could instantly judge who was coming toward them and move to get out of the way.

When he wanted something, nonverbal Vincent always guided his partner's hand to the object without so much as a glance at the partner. In the pool, however, he clung tightly to his mother and looked at her desperately when asked to stand up in the water on his own.

The following section provides strategies for tailoring tasks to a child's individual learning modes, motivation, and skills. This is followed by a summary of the possible functions of eye contact. Finally, task sequences for developing awareness and eye contact according to the various instruction paradigms are described.

Key Questions for Evaluating a Child's Skills

Attention and eye contact incorporate diverse abilities, such as being aware of other people, reacting to noises and movement, and looking at people when being addressed. We share events and feelings with others, but also—at a much more sophisticated level—we call attention to ourselves and interpret the glances of others (Quill, 2002).

To teach eye contact, the therapist must understand the abilities of the individual child with ASD. For example, is the child aware of other children or adults? Some children ignore the existence of other people, such as the child who runs into others in the playground. Other children stand at the edge of groups and withdraw from social contact. One may observe brief eye contact, watching from the corner of the eye and pausing when being addressed, in these children. In all cases, it is important to establish whether the child is able to communicate wishes, requests, protests, anxieties, joy, surprise, and so forth, and couple them with attention and eye contact.

Even if the child is not able to do so, his or her wish to be given a favorite item, request for help to open the candy jar, or anxiety at not being able to feel the bottom of the swimming pool may motivate him or her to look at his or her interaction partner. Key strategies for successful eye contact and attention training, therefore, involve the situations in which the child is motivated to communicate or respond to events. The answers to the following questions may provide a starting place for developing strategies that motivate a child into making eye contact.

Questions that help determine the best way for a child to learn

- Does the child respond with awareness or eye contact to noises, movement, instructions, or calling?
- For what actions does the child need help (e.g., opening a container, grasping)?
- What series of actions are motivating for the child (e.g., eating, bouncing)?
- In what situations does the child display joy, curiosity, wonder, defensiveness, or anxiety?
- Does the child follow another person's pointing?
- Does the child establish eye contact or follow a gaze spontaneously?
- What types of actions lead to the child's spontaneous eye contact (e.g., romping, tickling, play)?
- Can the child attract the attention of others?

In developing tasks to establish joint attention, therapists should incorporate the child's prerequisite skills, preferred learning channels, interests, and motivation.

DEVELOPMENTAL LEVELS FOR EYE CONTACT TRAINING

Typically developing children can look at their interaction partners as early as at 3 months of age. Even before 8 months of age, some children can direct their gaze to an object their mother is looking at or communicate nonverbally by looking at interesting or desired objects and then at the interaction partner (Kiphard, 1996; Wing, 1988).

Desires, requests, aversions, commentary, and questions can be communicated even before a child has learned her or his first words. For example, an infant looks from a barking dog to her mother and asks by her gaze whether the dog is a threat. This joint attention is developed in several stages and includes functions that also are found later in verbal communication.

For children with ASD, sequences and strategies for training attention and eye contact are not easy to define. While some children respond to massed trials of "look at me," others need general training in localizing noises, hearing their name, or responding to a gesture. Some children learn to establish eye contact more easily in rough-play sessions or through the peekaboo game than with traditional therapy drills. Hiding a child's eyes behind his hands, a blanket, a cushion, or furniture, coupled with sung repetitions of "Peekaboo—Where are you?," not only encourages children to establish eye contact and smile, but also invites them to initiate this game (Gutstein & Sheely, 2002; Twachtman-Cullen, 2004).

A child who brings an object to a person must have both the person and the object in sight. "Bring the newspaper to daddy" and similar exercises prepare a child for social awareness. To teach a child that eye contact can express a desire, a parent or therapist can hold a favorite object at his or her eye level. The child receives the object when he or she looks at the therapist. This exercise is relatively easy and can be performed in therapy or everyday situations.

It is more difficult to train eye contact for situations in which the child needs help or expresses surprise to the interaction partner, such as when a radio-controlled car moves. For the child to learn this type of eye contact, the therapist may need to first train the child to follow the therapist's finger with her or his gaze. This behavior is automatic for typically developing children, but many children with ASD need special training to learn it. Making the behavior automatic so the child is able to follow pointing gestures on a visit to the zoo (see Figure 7.1), for example, also requires special training. The speed exercises included in the precision teaching example later aims for automaticity in following pointing.

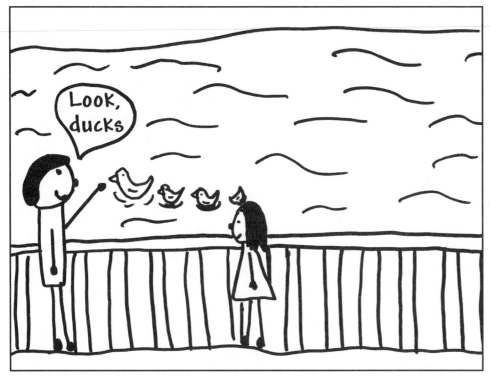

FIGURE 7.1. Children with ASD often need specific instructions to follow a pointing gesture.

To attract the attention of their interaction partners, nonverbal children must be able to alert partners to pictures, word cards, hand signs, or physical expression. The children must first notice that the partner does not look at them and get his attention by getting closer, touching him, showing their pictures, or even vocalizing.

As training progresses, more difficult objectives can be set, such as asking the child to discern what a partner wants from the direction in which he or she is looking. Does the child understand that a picture of a smiley face is "looking" at a can of Sprite and not at the gummy bears favored by the child (see Figure 7.2)? Joint attention is an early precursor to understanding the motivations of others and developing empathy.

TRAINING SEQUENCE FOR ATTENTION, EYE CONTACT, AND JOINT ATTENTION

The following list summarizes the training sequence of tasks for attention, eye contact, and joint attention:

> To give attention
> When called or addressed
> As request for
>> Person
>> Object
>> Action
>> Help

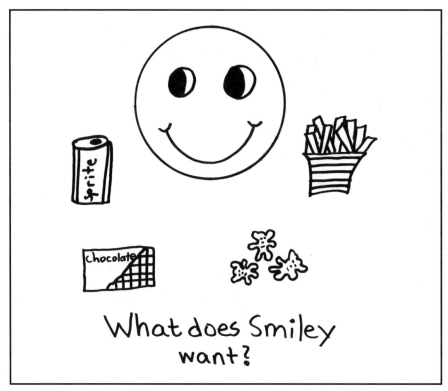

FIGURE 7.2. The child must be taught to observe others' wishes by following their eye gaze. In this exercise, the therapist says, "What does Smiley want?"

As expression of
    Greeting
    Parting
    Surprise
    Joy
    Anxiety
To question
    "What is it?"
    "Where is it?"
    "Who has it?"
As spontaneous directed gaze
To follow pointing

The following section examines these training topics in more detail.

Readiness to learn is closely related to the ability to pause, look, and listen. With most children with ASD, general attention training must be incorporated at the start of the STEP training. Children must learn to pause and pay attention to noises, movements, their name being called, and simple commands, such as "Look." Intensive exercises with clear instructions, guidance, and reinforcement have proven successful for many children with ASD.

To Give Attention

At the start of therapy, some children with ASD attend for no more than a few seconds. The concentration span is increased progressively by assigning simple tasks, such as matching, and using effective reinforcers. Initially, short periods of attention, such as 5 minutes, are sufficient. As the therapy progresses, the attention span is increased to 20 to 30 minutes. Providing predictable task sequences as well as breaks for physical activity often helps to increase the number of tasks the child can complete. Most children with ASD, even those who are very restless, have learned to become attentive within a week in the STEP program.

> Visitors to the STEP program often noted that students were very attentive and motivated to learn. This basic skill was developed by intense attention training and usually accomplished within the first week.

Later, children learn to attract the attention of an interaction partner. For example, in the PECS program, children are taught initially to approach the partner from progressively increasing distances and give him or her the requested picture or word card (Bondy & Frost, 1994). As training progresses, the therapist deliberately turns away from the child so that he or she must gain the therapist's attention by physical contact or turning the therapist's head to see the card. In early attention exercises, unexpected noises, such as musical instruments, an alarm clock, a barking dog, or a radio-controlled car or animal, or gestures can be used to elicit attention.

When Called or Addressed

Some children with ASD respond positively to frequent repetition of instructions such as "Look at me." Combining this instruction with the therapist's pointing to his or her eyes can usually develop eye contact. The therapist may also want to hold interesting objects in front of his or her eyes. More subtle cues, such as interrupting the child's activity until he looks, can also trigger eye contact.

As Request for People, Objects, or Actions

One approach to teaching eye contact that often motivates the child is to interrupt behavior chains such as climbing stairs, bouncing on a lap or trampoline, or eating a favorite meal (Goetz et al., 1985). The interaction partner interrupts these actions until the child looks at the partner. Happy, spontaneous looking often can be observed during the training.

As Request for Help

A child can also be motivated to look at the interaction partner to ask for help, such as when a favorite candy or toy is in a transparent but closed container that the child cannot open independently.

As Expression of Greeting or Parting

Play-based exercises are often helpful in teaching children to make eye contact in arrival or departure situations. Repeated scripts such as, "Knock, knock, who's there?," "Hello," and "Bye-bye" at doors or with dolls or puppets are often fun to practice for therapist and child.

As Expression of Feelings

In a recent study, my colleagues and I showed that young children with ASD look in the same direction as the interaction partner when unfamiliar noises or sights, such as laughing mirrors (i.e., party mirrors in which movement activates giggling) or bouncing spiders, are presented (Tan & Bernard-Opitz, 2002). Parents often report that their children have good eye contact when they are tickled or engaged in sensorimotor activities. Because sharing feelings is an essential function of eye contact, situations that elicit positive feelings are useful in eye contact training. Romping on the bed with parents or with friends at play, tickling, hiding, or catching games prompt an exchange of joyful eye contact among many children with ASD.

To Question

A typical child would probably ask, "What's that?" or "What's rattling in the box?" if a remote-controlled object was suddenly activated in a closed box. For a nonverbal child with autism, unfamiliar situations can be planned deliberately to prompt questioning eye contact.

As Spontaneous Directed Gaze

Another important method of establishing eye contact is by creating opportunities (Goetz et al., 1985). Obstacles and unexpected emotional events can be planned deliberately to encourage the child to communicate spontaneously. A child who finds a sock in her lunchbox instead of the expected treat may give a look of protest or question. The long-term objective of the joint attention tasks already described is to promote the child's looking in a given direction spontaneously.

To Follow Pointing

Initially, attractive objects such as bubbles or balloons can be used to teach the child to follow the direction of a pointing finger (e.g., "Look at the bubbles!"). As the exercise progresses, however, the child also learns to direct his attention to things that are neutral or uninteresting. At the same time, the verbal instruction can be changed from pointing out the object (e.g., "Look at the bird") to asking questions (e.g., "What is that?" "What do you see?"). In precision teaching programs, these instructions are progressively given more quickly to automate the response of looking where the finger is pointing.

Methods To Develop Eye Contact To Express Wishes and To Question

Similar to the above strategies are *communicative temptations* (Wetherby & Prizant, 1993). In this approach, actions such as blowing bubbles, unwrapping chocolate, or peeling a banana are carried out in slow motion. Obstacles are then introduced or surprises planned to encourage communication and to prompt the child to comment. The following situations, adapted from Wetherby and Prizant (1993) and Tan and Bernard-Opitz (2002), are helpful in triggering eye contact associated with the functions of requesting, pausing, commenting, naming, and questioning.

Situation	Example
Requesting	• Give the child a tightly closed container with some of her or his favorite reinforcers in it. • Place the child's favorite reinforcers out of reach. • Offer the child an object and pull it away playfully when he or she reaches for it. • Stop the ball in the middle of a game of catch. • Prevent the child from playing by holding her or his hands.
Pausing, Commenting, Naming, Questioning	• Make an unexpected noise. • Put on an interesting mask. • Operate a new toy. • "Accidentally" spill or tip over a fruit basket. • Offer a picture book. • Place a vibrating toy in the child's hand. • Put a noisemaker or vibrating object in a closed box. • Hide an interesting object in one hand and offer both hands closed to the child. • Program an electronic vehicle to make various maneuvers. • Activate a musical comb as you comb the child's hair.

TRAINING PROGRAM OVERVIEW

Form 7.1 outlines training programs to develop attention, eye contact, and joint attention skills. The listed teaching targets should be assessed prior to the intervention and following a period

Form 7.1. Overview of the STEP training programs for attention, eye contact, and joint attention; can be used as a pretest and posttest.

STEP Training Overview:
Attention, Eye Contact, and Joint Attention

Child _____ Teacher _____

❐ Pretest ❐ Posttest

Attention, Eye Contact, and Joint Attention Skill	Task	Date Tested	Child's Response +	Child's Response −	Notes
To give attention					
When called or addressed					
As request for					
Person					
Object					
Action					
Help					
As expression of					
Greeting					

of training. Once the child's profile of skills, learning channels, and interests has been determined, the therapist can select one of the four subsequent teaching methods. A reproducible copy of the form can be found in Appendix 7.A.

EXAMPLE TASKS: DISCRETE TRIAL FORMAT

Example Task I: Attention

- Child and therapist sit facing one another.
- The therapist says, "Get ready," and guides the child's hands to the side of his or her chair or the table surface.
- If the child imitates the movement within 3 seconds, she or he is praised and receives a small reinforcer.
- If not, the therapist places the child's hands in the position that was demonstrated.
- The exercise is repeated 10 times.

Example Task 2: Look at Therapist Upon Command

- Child and therapist sit facing one another.
- Every 5 to 10 seconds, the child is told, "Look at me."
- If the child looks at the therapist within 2 seconds, for at least 1 second, she or he is praised and receives a small reinforcer.
- If the child responds after 2 seconds or not at all, the therapist looks away briefly and begins a new trial.
- The exercise is repeated 10 times.

Note. The therapist can facilitate guiding the child's gaze to the therapist's eyes by pointing to his or her eyes with the index and middle fingers or by holding up a small reinforcer to his or her eyes. If a child fails to benefit from massed trial teaching of eye contact, alternative methods should be attempted, such as interrupting routines.

Form 7.2 shows how these examples could be recorded using the blank data form for discrete trial format in Appendix 7.B.

Related Literature

Lovaas, O. I. (1981). *Teaching developmentally disabled children: The me book*. Austin, TX: PRO-ED.

Maurice, C., Green, G., & Luce, S. C. (1996). *Behavioral intervention for young children with autism*. Austin, TX: PRO-ED.

EXAMPLE TASKS: PRECISION TEACHING

Example Task I: Look at People in a Circle

- A number of people (adults or children) stand or sit in a circle around the child.
- The child is instructed to offer each person her or his hand and to look at the person.
- The instruction can also be related to eye contact or greeting ("Look over here!" "Say, 'hello'"). See Figure 7.3.
- The therapist counts the number of times the child responds with eye contact within a 30-second period.

Form 7.2. Example data form for discrete trial format method of teaching attention, eye contact, and joint attention skills.

Data Form for Discrete Trial

Child _____   Teacher _____

Skill Area ___Attention, Eye Contact, and Joint Attention___

In addition to recording the child's performance, indicate specifics about the task setup, sc
schedule. Try to conduct about 10 trials per date and five sessions per week. Note that if the
Plot data on daily learning graphs.

Target Skill	Task Setup		Prompt	Consequence
	Material or Task	**Instruction**		
Attention		"Get ready"	Show and guide the child's hands over the sides of the chair	Verbal and material reinforcement
When called or addressed		"Look at me"	Guide the gaze with the finger	Verbal and material reinfor...

- The goal is to increase the frequency of eye contact in each subsequent drill.
- If there is an incorrect response, or none at all, the therapist or interaction partner redirects the child's gaze.

Prerequisite
The child already must have learned to look at different people when asked to do so.

Variations
- The number of people and speed of the greeting are increased successively until the child has reached a predetermined level.
- Later, the child is instructed, through role play or written or pictured sequences, as to whom she or he should greet (e.g., the person she or he is looking at) and whom she or he should not greet.
- The exercise may be conducted with the child's playmates or siblings.

Example Task 2: Look in the Direction of Pointing Finger

- The child and the therapist sit on the floor surrounded by various toys or objects.
- The therapist instructs the child to look at the toy or object at which the therapist is pointing.
- Once the child has mastered this, the therapist points to different toys or objects in rapid succession.
- The therapist tells the child, "Look over here," when starting the trial.
- The therapist counts the number of object eye contacts in a 30-second period.
- If the child makes an incorrect response, or none at all, his or her gaze is redirected to the object indicated.
- The goal is to increase the number of times the child looks in the direction requested in each subsequent drill until the child has reached the predetermined level.

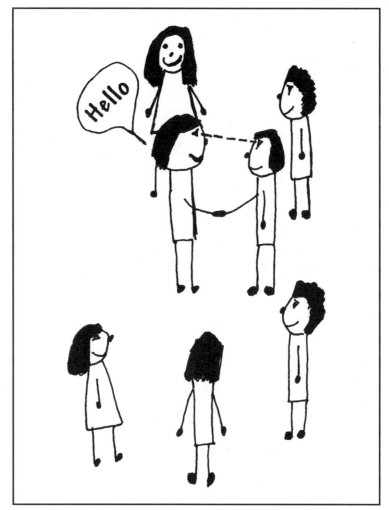

FIGURE 7.3. Repetitive greeting of different people can enhance spontaneous eye contact.

Prerequisite
The child must already have learned to look at various objects to which the therapist points.

Variation
The speed of the instructions, number of objects, and their distance from the child are progressively increased.

Note. The expected frequency standard for this type of "See–Do" exercise with autistic children is 35 to 50 responses per minute (Fabrizio & Moors, 2003). At this rate, stability of the behavior is likely. However, individual deviations from this learning objective should also be taken into account. The rate at which the behavior of an individual child is stable and generalized should be assessed and confirmed (Leach, Coyle, & Cole, 2003).

Form 7.3 shows how these examples could be recorded using the blank data form for precision teaching in Appendix 7.B.

Related Literature

Fabrizio, M. A., & Moors, A. L. (2003). Evaluating mastery: Measuring instructional outcomes for children with autism. *European Journal of Behavior Analysis, 4,* 23–36.

Leach, D., Coyle, C. A., & Cole, P. G. (2003). Fluency in the classroom. In R. F. Waugh (Ed.), *On the forefront of educational psychology.* New York: Nova Science.

Form 7.3. Example data form for precision teaching of attention, eye contact, and joint attention skills.

	Task Setup				Le
Target Skill	**Material or Task**	**Instruction**	**Time Unit**	**Consequence**	H
As expression of greeting or parting	Look at people in circle	"Say, 'hello'"	Frequency of directed gaze in 30 seconds	Nodding confirmation after every time and tokens every time number of correct responses increases	Se
To follow pointing	Look in direction of finger pointing at various objects	"Look here"	Number of eye-object contacts in 30 seconds		Se

Data Form for Precision Te...

Child _____   Teacher _____

Skill Area ___Attention, Eye Contact, and Joint Attention_____

EXAMPLE TASKS: NATURAL AND EXPERIENCE-BASED TEACHING

Example Task 1: Request for Person and Expression of Surprise or Joy

- The therapist gently hides the child's eyes with the therapist's hands.
- The therapist says or sings, "Peekaboo, where are you?"
- The therapist removes her or his hands at the syllable "boo" and again at the word "you."
- If the child makes eye contact, the therapist praises the child and reinforces through tickling, stroking, blowing on skin, and so on.

Variation

- Some children respond better if they cover the therapist's eyes with their hands.
- This game can also be played with cloths, play tunnels, doors, and so forth.

Example Task 2: Request for Favorite Object or Action

- The child eats a favorite food, such as ice cream, with a spoon.
- The therapist says, "Eating ice cream—mmm" about three times.
- The therapist then briefly prevents the child from putting the spoon in her or his mouth.
- The child is allowed to continue eating when she or he looks at the therapist.
- The child is praised for eye contact with "Yes, good. Eat the ice cream."
- If the child does not look at the therapist, the therapist briefly holds the ice cream in front of her or his face so that the child looks into the therapist's eyes.

Variation

Other activities the therapist could interrupt include climbing stairs, rocking, bouncing on a trampoline, filling the bathtub, playing in the sandbox, and so forth.

Example Task 3: Request for Help

- The child is given a tightly closed glass container with a favorite object inside.
- The therapist instructs the child to make eye contact with the therapist.
- When eye contact is made successfully, the therapist offers to help the child open the container.

Variations

- Objects the child wants are placed out of reach.
- When the child tries to reach them by moving the therapist's hand, the therapist asks the child to make eye contact.
- When the child makes eye contact successfully, the therapist retrieves the object.

Table 7.1 provides examples of how natural teaching can be used to develop attention skills. Form 7.4 shows a data form that can be used to record a child's responses to natural teaching. This form can be reproduced from Appendix 7.B.

Related Literature

Gutstein, S. E., & Sheely, R. K. (2002). *Relationship development intervention with young children*. London: Jessica Kingsley.

EXAMPLE TASKS: VISUAL LEARNING

Example Task 1: Eye Contact with Person Calling

- The child and the therapist sit a small distance apart.
- Every so often, the therapist calls the child's name clearly but soothingly. For children who lack the required language skills, the therapist waves.

Form 7.4. Blank data form for natural and experience-based teaching of attention, eye contact, and joint attention skills.

Data Form for Natural and Experience

Child _____ Teacher _____

Skill Area ___Attention, Eye Contact, and Joint Attention___

Target Skill	Task Setup		Consequence
	Material or Task	**Instruction**	

Table 7.1

**Examples of Ways Natural and Experience-Based Teaching
Can Be Used To Develop Attention, Eye Contact, and Joint Attention**

Attention, Eye Contact, and Joint Attention Skill	Examples
To give attention	Interesting noises are made or remote-controlled toys are activated from various places, and the child's attention is directed to them (e.g., rustling of chips bag or chocolate wrapper, alarm clock, musical instruments).
When called or addressed	The child is called by different people or from various locations. He or she is praised for each correct response and receives a natural reinforcer (e.g., outdoor shoes, water in the bathtub and bathing).
As request for	
Person	Peekaboo games are played by hiding the child's or therapist's eyes with hands or with blankets, cushions, furniture, and so forth.
Action	The therapist comments continuously while feeding the child: "Food, mmmm," and interrupts until the child looks at the therapist.
Object	Attractive objects are placed in a closed glass container. The therapist does not open the container until the child establishes eye contact.
As expression of	
Greeting Parting	Greeting and parting are practiced at a door or curtain or with a puppet theater. Recurring scripts such as, "Knock-knock—hello!" are combined with the opening of the door or curtain. The child is praised for making eye contact.
Surprise	A clockwork musical toy (e.g., jack-in-the-box) is wound slowly and stopped shortly before the lid springs open. When it does open, the therapist makes a sound of surprise to prompt the child to make eye contact.
Joy Anxiety	The child is placed in a situation that causes him or her joy or *mild* anxiety, such as being lifted into the air, rocked, or led into a darkened room. The therapist waits for the child to make eye contact before lifting the child higher, putting down the child, or switching on the light.
As question	
"What is it?"	The child's hand is placed in a container or grab bag filled with Styrofoam and objects of various consistencies, surfaces, shapes, weights, and noises. Before the child pulls her or his hand out, the therapist asks, "What is that?" and attempts to establish eye contact with the child.
"Where is it?"	The therapist blows up a balloon and lets it go. The therapist watches the balloon and instructs the child to watch it too.
"Who has it?"	One of two or more interaction partners hides an interesting object behind his or her back. The child must find out where the object is hidden by looking at the correct partner.
As spontaneous directed gaze	The therapist blocks the child's path and does not get out of the way until the child looks at him or her. Spontaneous eye contact is praised.
To follow pointing	During routine activities, interesting things are pointed out to the child. The therapist directs the child's gaze to the object or actions at which the finger is pointing.

- If the child looks at the therapist, the child receives a small reward.
- If not, the therapist moves into the child's field of vision and tries to attract her or his attention.

Variations
- The therapist moves progressively farther away from the child.
- The therapist calls from different locations.
- Different people call from different locations. The child must look at the person who is calling or waving to him or her.

Example Task 2: Eye Contact with Object and Person

- The child plays a game that he or she enjoys, such as bouncing on the trampoline.
- The therapist tells the child or makes a gesture or signal to "Bounce."
- The therapist accompanies this verbally, saying, "Bounce, bounce, bounce ..."
- The therapist occasionally gives a clear instruction or sign to "Stop," such as holding a hand up.
- The child should anticipate the instruction or sign and turn to look the therapist in the eyes.

Example Task 3: Eye Contact as Question About Location of an Object

- The therapist hides an important part of a favorite game (e.g., piece of jigsaw puzzle) in her or his hand.
- When the child reaches for it, the therapist holds on to it until the child looks at the therapist.
- The therapist may find it helpful to hold the game piece up to her or his eyes.
- The therapist returns the game piece to the child when she or he makes eye contact.

Form 7.5 shows how these examples could be recorded using the blank data form for visual learning in Appendix 7.B.

Form 7.5. Example data form for visual learning method of teaching attention, eye contact, and joint attention skills.

Data Form for Visual Lea

Child _____   Teacher _____

Skill Area ___Attention, Eye Contact, and Joint Attention___

Target Skill	Task	Instruction	
		Verbal	**Visual**
When called or addressed	The child should respond to waving or hearing her or his name called.	"(Name), look."	Wave
As request for action	The child is allowed to continue with activity (e.g., bouncing on trampoline) after making eye contact	"Bounce, bounce, bounce," followed by clear "Stop!"	Sign for trampoline and gesture for "bounce" followed by clear "Stop!" signal
As question	Therapist puts a jig-	"Where is the puzzle	Sign for jigsaw

Related Literature

A basic dictionary of American Sign Language terms. (n.d.). Retreived July 3, 2006, from
    http://www.masterstech-home.com/ASLDict.html

Boswell, S. (2005). *TEACCH preschool curriculum guide.* Chapel Hill, NC: Division TE-
    ACCH, University of North Carolina at Chapel Hill.

Quill, K. A. (2002). *Do, watch, listen, say.* Baltimore: Brookes.

Schopler, E., Lansing, M. D., & Waters, L. (1982). *Teaching activities for autistic children:
    Vol. III. Individualized assessment and treatment for autistic and developmentally dis-
    abled children.* Austin, TX: PRO-ED.

Matching and Sorting

Section Overview

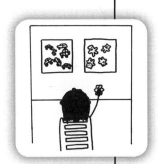

IMPORTANCE OF MATCHING AND SORTING

Matching and sorting are important skills for the development of thinking, language, and problem solving. Typically developing children learn to distinguish colors, shapes, sizes, amounts, and categories while completing puzzles and shape-sorters, putting toys back into the correct storage containers, placing trains on tracks and cars into garages, placing doll furniture into different rooms of a dollhouse, selecting the right pencils for pencil cases, and putting groceries into the relevant compartments of a refrigerator. Even before an infant can request "milk" or "drink," she knows that the rubber nipple goes onto the bottle and that the milk carton is in the refrigerator, which can only be found in the kitchen.

What Is the Difference Between Matching and Sorting?

Matching entails putting an object with another identical or similar object (e.g., a cup with a cup), or with the other half of a pair (e.g., a knife with a fork). *Sorting,* on the other hand, refers to separating a number of objects according to categories or types (e.g., the child is asked to separate some pencils, bricks, and cars into three groups) or putting objects into some kind of order (e.g., organizing objects according to their size). *Note:* In therapy sessions, the word *match* is frequently used, even when the task is sorting.

Why are matching and sorting skills important?

- Comprehension of sameness, similarity, and difference
- Comprehension of belonging pairs, associations, and categories
- Comprehension of concepts such as color, shape, size, letters, numbers, and amounts
- Comprehension of reinforcement for correct responses
- Development of language and communication
- Generalization

For many children with ASD, however, the world is not as well organized as a kitchen with milk in the refrigerator. Only through systematic training of matching then sorting do they comprehend which objects belong together, which form concepts, and which are included under one name. The children's difficulty is such that they may associate the word *dog* only with their neighbor's poodle, but not the Doberman one street away or the toy dog on the shelf in their own room. This does not mean that the poodle, the Doberman, and the toy dog should all be brought together to teach the concept. Instead, photos or schematic drawings of different kinds of dogs can be matched to various representatives in the category.

In his therapy session, 10-year-old Daniel always received a small piece of snack sausage for signing the word *sausage.* However, his parents indicated that he had not generalized the sign to home. Only after sorting various kinds of sausages was Daniel able to recognize that the liver sausage used at home also was a sausage.

Many children with ASD have excellent visual and spatial skills. They are exceptionally capable of completing puzzles and always know where Mom has hidden their beloved alphabet letters. Even in intricate parking lots, they know exactly where the family car is parked. They remember directions after only one drive and often insist, vehemently, on taking the same route. Many of these visual children, however, can sort an object only by its visual features and not by its associated function.

Five-year-old Annie was able to sort colors, shapes, letters, and numbers, but consistently put oranges with balls instead of with other food items such as bananas. Obviously the fact that an orange was round like a ball was more significant to her than the fact that it was a fruit.

KEY QUESTIONS FOR EVALUATING A CHILD'S SKILLS

By observing a child doing everyday tasks, the therapist can gain an impression of whether the child's skills are visual or conceptual. Such observations provide a window into the child's strengths and weaknesses and should be considered when developing useful teaching targets and therapy methods. Consider the following questions:

Questions to determine the best way for a child to learn

Is the child able to:

- stack plastic drinking cups?
- stack or line up blocks?
- put the correct shapes into the correct holes of a shape sorter?
- complete puzzles? If so, how many pieces?
- identify his or her shoes?
- match colored socks?
- sort a selection of objects (e.g., all pencils together, all cars together)?
- sort objects according to color or size?
- recognize the family car?
- find the family car in a parking lot?
- find liked items at home or in a supermarket?
- match items that belong together (e.g., lids to containers)?
- recognize packages of food (e.g., familiar cereal)?
- recognize pictures, logos, or written words (e.g., traffic or restroom sign)?
- match photos of people with the real people?
- match photos that show the same emotional expressions?
- put objects back where they belong?

DEVELOPMENTAL LEVELS FOR MATCHING AND SORTING SKILLS

Many typically developing 18-month-old toddlers already know where everyday objects are kept. They are able to sort simple objects into categories and return items to where they belong. At the age of 2 years, they can usually match at least two objects to a corresponding picture, in addition to matching two colors, shapes, and sizes (Kiphard, 1996). At the age of 3 years, children can sort all colors, shapes, sizes, and pictures.

Many children with ASD exhibit age-appropriate or even advanced skills in completing puzzles or matching tasks such as required on the nonverbal *Leiter International Performance Scale* (Roid & Miller, 1997). These children demonstrate good visual–spatial differentiation. Tasks like these, which have a clear structure, are often motivating for children with ASD. They can move from completing simple inset puzzles of common objects, shapes, or colors to working on jigsaw puzzles with four or more pieces. Some young children with ASD can even put together highly complex interlocking puzzles without any training.

While typical preschool children tend to match objects before matching pictures, many children with ASD find it easier to work with pictures than with objects. Some of these children can even match letters, numbers, amounts, abstract symbols, or word cards before they can master picture matching. Children with ASD also may have a harder time matching items to categories because they do not have the required language concepts. Tasks such as sorting by category and matching pictures of people and emotional expressions are often relevant learning targets for these children.

Although the developmental sequence presented below provides a suggested sequence for training targets, the final selection of goals should be individualized and matched to the prerequisites and interests of the child and her or his social context. The choice of whether to carry out the training with real objects or with photos, schematics, or line drawings can mean the difference between fast or slow progress for the child.

Typical Sequence of Difficulty for Matching and Sorting Skills

Least Difficult

- Inserting objects into another of the same kind, such as plastic cups
- Matching identical objects placed next to each other, without a distracter
- Matching identical objects placed next to each other, with one distracter
- Sorting identical objects into sets, each set with its own container; start with two sets, with two objects in each set (later, more objects in each set)
- Matching belonging pairs
- Classifying objects into two (later, three or four) categories
- Inserting 4 (later, 6 or 10) cutout puzzle pieces
- Assembling an interlocking puzzle
- Matching objects to pictures and pictures to objects
- Matching and sorting colors, shapes, and sizes
- Matching and sorting numbers, letters, and word cards
- Matching and sorting amounts, such as pictures of one, two, and three apples
- Matching same or similar pictures of people
- Matching pictures of people with similar emotional expressions

Most Difficult

- Putting everyday objects back to their original location (e.g., shoe in shoe rack, pot on stove, CD into CD stand)

HOW TO CONDUCT THE TRAINING

When matching and sorting items using the *discrete trial format* of teaching, therapist and child usually sit across the table from each other. Sorting trays or colored mats indicate where the child is supposed to put the items. A typical matching task may be taught as follows:

Step 1. Hand the child an object such as a plastic plate, requesting that it be put with another identical one, which is already on the table. The child needs to stack 8 to 10 plates in this manner. The criterion to be met for this plate-stacking task is 9 or 10 out of 10 trials (90%–100%) completed correctly at one time or 8 out of 10 trials (80%) on 2 consecutive days.

Step 2. Repeat the original task but add a distracting item, such as a cup. It can be placed at a distance of about 3 inches from the plate. The position of plate and cup should be varied randomly to prevent the child from fixating on one position.

Step 3. Once the plate is consistently discriminated from a distracter, cups can be added as stimuli the child has to discriminate. Plates and cups are handed to the child in blocks of three, meaning that a cup is given to the child three times in succession followed by three plates in succession. Once the child has mastered about six to eight items, he or she can start Step 4.

Step 4. In this step, children learn to match and sort similar items, such as different-colored cups, before going on to other categories, such as dishes.

The *precision teaching* method assumes that learning is not an even process, but one where the first learning steps take much longer than the ones that follow. While learning to match the first two items may take a week, the child usually masters future tasks much faster. To picture this exponential increase in the number of correct responses over time, proponents of this method suggest therapists prepare a logarithmic presentation of correct and incorrect responses. These celeration charts display the child's progress over days, weeks, and months. The last response of the child, as well as group norms, constitutes the objective for the coming task. While research studies have made initial findings on fluency rates in different learning channels (Fabrizio & Moors, 2003), these have to be considered preliminary. The main question for fluency criteria is whether reached performance guarantees generalization to new tasks. An example would be whether reading one text according to fluency standards predicts the performance on another text (Leach et al., 2003). Concrete steps in conducting the training are summarized in the precision teaching examples later in this section.

Sorting tasks that follow the model of *natural and experience-based learning* tend to be less structured and more embedded into everyday activities. Does the child know where things are and where to keep them? Does she or he know that blocks should be stacked or put into a pattern and not be inserted into a CD player? Does she or he know that knives and forks belong in the sorting tray in the drawer and that cushions usually go on the sofa or the chair? Is she or he able to recognize grandparents, siblings, or parents in a photo album, even though they are pictured in different clothes and at different ages? If the answer to any of these kinds of questions is *no,* then the therapist should make use of the situations to teach the concepts whenever possible.

For *visual learning,* following the TEACCH model or pictured activity sequences, it is important that matching and sorting tasks have a clear arrangement and a predictable ending. Working in one direction (from left to right) and placing completed tasks into a "finish box" make this format easy for children to understand. Independent performance is a core goal within this teaching method (Mesibov & Howley, 2003).

Training Program Overview

Form 7.6 outlines training programs to develop matching and sorting skills. The listed teaching targets should be assessed prior to the intervention and following a period of training. Once the child's profile of skills, learning channels, and interests has been determined, the therapist can select one of the four subsequent teaching methods. A reproducible copy of the form can be found in Appendix 7.A.

Form 7.6. Overview of the STEP training programs for matching and sorting skills; can be used as a pretest and posttest.

STEP Training Overview:
Matching and Sorting

Child _____ Teacher _____

❏ Pretest   ❏ Posttest

Matching and Sorting Skill	Materials (circle those tested)	Date Tested	Child's Response		Other Materials Tested
			+	−	

Identical objects	Dishes and utensils
	  Cups, plates, bowls
	  Spoons, forks, knives
	Toys
	  Duplo or Lego blocks
	  Cars, ping-pong balls
	School and office supplies
	  Pencils, papers, cards
	  Paper clips
	Clothing
	  Shoes, socks
	Other:				

Objects that belong	Dishes and utensils				

Example Tasks: Discrete Trial Teaching

Example Task 1: Matching Identical Objects

- Child and therapist sit facing each other.
- On the table in front of them is a plastic cup, right side up or upside down.
- The therapist holds a second cup at the child's eye level and says, "Match with same (or stack or put in or put together or where does it go?)."
- Once the child has responded correctly, she or he is praised and receives a reinforcer.
- If the child fails to respond or responds incorrectly (e.g., throws the cup), a prompt is given using the least-restrictive method first (In order: pointing, distance prompt, errorless prompt, physical guidance).
- The task is repeated 10 times.

Note

For children with fine-motor problems, putting identical objects such as beads or bears into a container may be easier than inserting items into small spaces and stacking (see Figure 7.4).

Variations

- Several cups can be arranged in rows of two or three such that the child can stack them.
- The task can be expanded to matching color, shape, and size.

Task Example 2: Matching Colors

- Child and therapist sit facing each other at a table.
- In front of the child are two small trays, each with a red toy and a yellow toy (e.g., two colored block towers, stringed beads, cars).

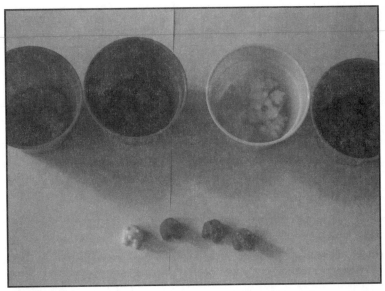

FIGURE 7.4. In this sorting task, the child places colored plastic bears into the cup with the other bears.

- The therapist holds up one of the toys at the child's eye level and says, "Match with same (or stack or put in or put together)."
- Once the child has matched the given object correctly, the therapist praises the child and says, "That's correct. This is red."
- If the child does not respond, the therapist points to the correct item or pushes the correct item closer as a prompt. If the child responds incorrectly, a prompt is used (see Example 1 for list).
- The task is repeated 10 times.

Notes
- The position of the trays is exchanged after about two trials.
- Discriminations are conducted in blocks of trials (e.g., blocks of five or three and random order).

Variations
- Different objects of one color, such as plastic spoons, cups, plates, pegs, and crayons, can be matched to a corresponding color tray.
- Colored tops of marker pens can be matched to the pen's color.
- Colored trays can be arranged in different ways, such as in rows of two or three.

Task Example 3: Matching Identical Pictures of People

- Child and therapist sit facing each other.
- On the table in front of them are four trays that have photos or schematic drawings or line drawings of a man, a woman, a girl, and a boy.
- Once the child attends, the therapist holds up a picture that matches one of those in the trays and says, "Match with same (or stack or put in or put together)."
- If the child matches correctly, the therapist praises and reinforces the child.
- The praise should incorporate the picture's label (e.g., "That's right. That is a man").
- If the child does not respond correctly, a prompt is used (see Example 1).
- The task is repeated 10 times.

Prerequisites
- The child must be able to match at least two pictures.
- Once the child is able to differentiate identical pictures, the therapist can introduce similar pictures.

Form 7.7. Example data form for discrete trial format method of teaching matching and sorting skills.

Data Form for Discrete Trial

Child _____   Teacher _____

Skill Area _Matching and Sorting_____

In addition to recording the child's performance, indicate specifics about the task setup, s
schedule. Try to conduct about 10 trials per date and five sessions per week. Note that if the
Plot data on daily learning graphs.

Target Skill	Task Setup		Prompt	Consequence
	Material or Task	**Instruction**		
Identical objects	10 plastic cups	"Match with same (or stack or put in)"	Physical guidance	Praise; reinforce
Colors	10 red and 10 yellow blocks	"Match with same (or put together or s	Pointing; distance prompt; physical guidance	"That's correct. This is red."

Variations

- Pictures that differ in size and quality can be used (color photos, black-and-white photos, drawings).
- Pictures can depict different ages, races, clothing, hairstyles, beards, and so forth.

Form 7.7 shows how these examples could be recorded using the blank data form for discrete trial format in Appendix 7.B.

Related Literature

Blank, M., McKirdy, L. S., & Payne, P. (2000). *Links to language.* Upper Montclair, NJ: HELP Associates.

Leaf, R., & McEachin, J. (1999). *A work in progress: Behavior management strategies and a curriculum for intensive behavioral treatment of autism.* New York: DLR Books.

Lovaas, O. I. (1981). *Teaching developmentally disabled children: The me book.* Austin, TX: PRO-ED.

Maurice, C., Green, G., & Luce, S. L. (1996). *Behavioral intervention for young children with autism.* Austin, TX: PRO-ED.

Partington, J. W., & Sundberg, M. L. (1998). *The assessment of basic language and learning skills.* Pleasant Hill, CA: Behavior Analysts.

EXAMPLE TASKS: PRECISION TEACHING

Example Task 1: Sorting Categories

- Child and therapist sit facing each other.
- On the table in front of them are two trays: one containing a toy animal and the other a toy car.

- The therapist hands the child a second animal or car and says, "Match (or put together or where does this go?)."
- Once the child has placed the item correctly, the therapist gives the child other objects and instructs, "Put as fast as you can."
- When the child sorts correctly, the therapist nods and intermittently praises the child.
- When the child sorts wrongly, the therapist quietly puts the wrongly placed object aside.
- The numbers of correct and incorrect responses within a 20-second period are counted.
- If the child has improved his or her previous performance, the therapist gives the child a Smiley.
- Once the child has three Smileys, he or she receives a reinforcer.

Variations

- Given a tray of unsorted cars and animals, the child sorts them into two categories independently, without instruction from the therapist.
- The child sorts toys into various categories (e.g., Lego and Duplo blocks, pencils, pens, crayons and markers, zoo, house, ocean animals).
- The therapist increases the number of categories.

Example Task 2: Matching Shapes and Sizes

- Show the child a worksheet with outline drawings of different basic shapes and sizes (see Figure 7.5).
- Give 4 (and later, up to 30) plastic chips or cardboard shapes that correspond to the shapes and sizes on the worksheet. The child is instructed to "Put with the same (or match or where does this go?)."
- Once the child has placed the item correctly, the therapist gives the child other objects and instructs, "Put as fast as you can."
- The numbers of correctly and incorrectly matched items within a 20-second period (later, 60-second period) are noted.
- Whenever the child improves his or her performance, he or she receives a reinforcer.

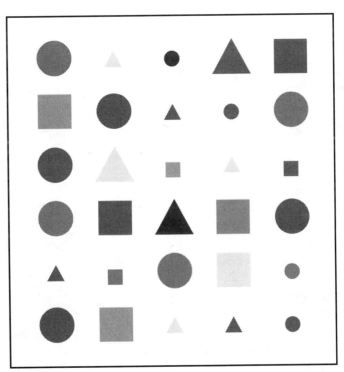

FIGURE 7.5. In this task, colored shapes and sizes have to be matched within a short time period.

Example Task 3: Matching Pictures of Emotional Expressions

- On the table there are 6 different emotion pictures arranged in a circle (see Figure 7.6).
- The therapist hands the child 10 identical pictures and instructs, "Put with same as fast as you can."
- When the child responds correctly, the therapist nods and intermittently praises.
- When the child matches wrongly, the therapist quietly puts the item to one side.
- The numbers of correctly and incorrectly matched items within a 20-second period (later, 30- and 60-second periods) are noted.
- When the child improves his or her previous performance, he or she receives a reinforcer.

Variations

- The child sorts a stack of pictures without any assistance.
- During the course of therapy, increase the task difficulty by making the emotional expressions less distinct.

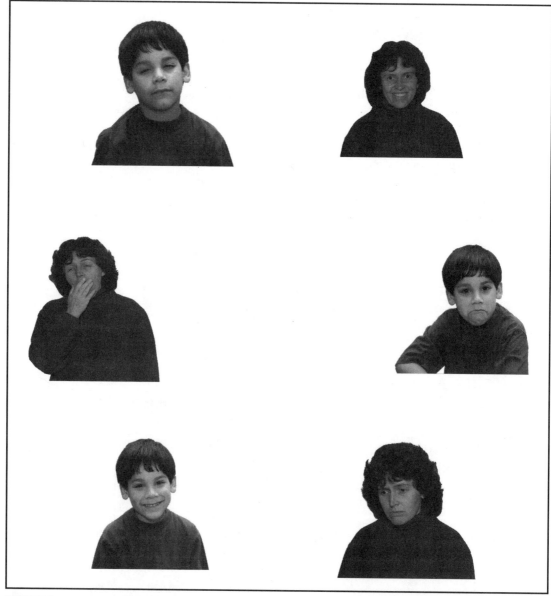

FIGURE 7.6. Here, the child matches photos of different emotional expressions. *Note.* Photos from *Picture This* [Computer software], by Silver Lining Multimedia, 2003, Peterborough, NH: Author. Copyright 2003 by Silver Lining Multimedia. Used with permission.

Note

See-do tasks such as these can be completed at a rate of 35 to 60 correct answers per minute (Fabrizio & Moors, 2003). Further research must be conducted to confirm whether these rates guarantee stable and generalized performance (see discussion by Leach et al., 2003).

Cross-Reference

Sorting tasks (see-do) can be complemented by tasks for language comprehension (hear-do), tasks for imitation (hear-say), and tasks for expressive language (see-say).

Form 7.8 shows how these examples could be recorded using the blank data form for precision teaching in Appendix 7.B.

Related Literature

Bondy, A., Dickey, D., & Buswell, S. (2002). *The pyramid approach to education: Lesson plans for young children.* Newark, DE: Pyramid Educational Products.

Fabrizio, M. A., & Moors, A. L. (2003). Evaluating mastery: Measuring instructional outcomes for children with autism. *European Journal of Behavior Analysis, 4,* 23–36.

Leach, D., Coyle, C. A., & Cole, P. G. (2003). Fluency in the classroom. In R. F. Waugh (Ed.), *On the forefront of educational psychology* (pp. 115–137). New York: Nova Science.

EXAMPLE TASKS: NATURAL AND EXPERIENCE-BASED LEARNING

Task Example 1: Matching Objects That Belong Together

- Child and therapist sit on the floor with a multistory toy parking garage housing some parked cars.
- The therapist hands the child a car and instructs, "Put it where it belongs."

Form 7.8. Example data form for precision teaching of matching and sorting skills.

Data Form for Precision Te

Child _____ Teacher _____

Skill Area ___Matching and Sorting_____

Target Skill	Task Setup		Time Unit	Consequence	Le H
	Material or Task	**Instruction**			
Categories	Toy animals and toy cars	"Match (or put together or Where does this go?)"	20 seconds		Se
Shapes	Worksheet with 30 shapes	"Put with same (or match or Where does this go?)"	20 seconds		Se
Emotions	10 pictures of emotio	"Put with same as fast as you	20 seconds		S

- The therapist praises the child for placing the car with the other vehicles and encourages her or him to drive a car down the ramp making engine sounds.

Variations

- At a later stage, the therapist offers vehicles that are too big for the garage or the ramp, to work on sizes or to differentiate rolling and nonrolling items.
- Have the child match marbles to a marble run or balls to a ball pool using functional reinforcers.
- Two, then later three and four, activities can be discriminated, such as putting Lego bricks onto a Lego board, toy people into a bus, and beads onto a string.

Task Example 2: Matching Objects that Belong Together and Storing Objects

- A variety of objects that belong in different locations are placed on the table or floor (e.g., pillows, pencils, books, videos, CDs, plates, hammers, teddy bears).
- The child is asked to "Put the things back where they belong."
- If the child responds correctly, the therapist praises the child and gives him or her functional reinforcers such as a dance with the teddy bear for putting him into his bed or a short pillow fight.
- If the child puts the object in the wrong place, the therapist models the correct placement and gives the child another chance with another item from the same category.

Note

At a beginning level, this task can be a simple matching task (e.g., At the stove, Mom asks, "Where does the lid go?"). At a more advanced stage, the child may need, for example, to clean up her or his room and find the belonging location for various objects scattered on the floor.

Prerequisite

The child should be able to recognize objects that go together.

Task Example 3: Completing Puzzles

- The child is shown a four-piece inset puzzle.
- The therapist puts three pieces in and asks the child to insert the last piece.
- The child is praised for responding correctly.
- The therapist empties the puzzle again and lets the child complete the last two pieces, continuing in this way until the child can put in all four pieces independently.

Variations

- Shape-, color-, and size-sorters, key boxes, or even regular keys are often motivating for children.
- Puzzle pieces with four straight edges are generally easier for beginners than puzzles with interlocking pieces. These can be constructed by cutting photos into two, four, and more same-size pieces and mounting them on cardboard.
- Puzzles come in various sizes, materials, and levels of difficulty. Puzzles with big knobs, floor puzzles, and puzzles from hardwood, rubber foam, or cardboard work well for children with ASD. Simple object inset puzzles with shapes, colors, sizes, numbers, and letters tend to be easier than puzzles with multiple interlocking pieces.

Cross-Reference

Objects that go together and puzzles with simple object pictures can also be used for language comprehension and expression.

Table 7.2 provides examples of how natural teaching can be used to develop matching and sorting skills. Form 7.9 shows a data form that can be used to record a child's responses to natural teaching. This form can be reproduced from Appendix 7.B.

Table 7.2
**Examples of Ways Natural and Experienced-Based Teaching
Can Be Used To Develop Matching and Sorting Skills**

Matching and Sorting Skill	Examples
Identical/similar objects	Toys
	Cars, blocks, tracks
	Everyday objects
	Books, audiotapes, videotapes, CDs
Objects that belong together	School supplies
	Pencils and pencil case
	Chalk or markers and chalkboard
	Sandwich and brown bag or sandwich box
	Office supplies
	Paper clips and container
	Letters and envelopes
	Envelopes and stamps
	Dishes and utensils
	Pot and lid
	Cup and saucer or plate
	Knife and fork
	Can and can opener
	Locations
	CD and CD player or computer
	Pillow and bed or sofa
	Milk and refrigerator
	Trash and trash can
Categories (Two or more items per category)	Toys
	Blocks
	Cars, trains
	Animals
	Dolls, puppets
	Groceries
	Food, drinks
	Vegetables, fruit
	Bread, muffins, bagels
	Cheese, bacon, ham
	Clothing
	Socks, shoes
	Pants, shorts, shirts
	Tools
	Screws, nuts, nails
	Hammers, screwdrivers
Puzzles	Inset puzzles with 1 to 4 pieces, later 10 or more
	Interlocking puzzles with 4 pieces, later 500 or more
Colors, shapes, sizes, lengths	Collect all objects of one color
	Sort socks by color or size
	Use shape-, size-, key-sorting boxes
	Match real keys to locks
	Match lids of various sizes to containers

(*continues*)

Table 7.2. *(Continued)*

Matching and Sorting Skill	Examples
Letters, words, numbers, amounts	Trace, draw, color, cut
	Match magnetic, play-dough letters, numbers, words
	Match letters in alphabet soup
	Set table for certain number of people
	Match number of dishes to family members
People	Sort photos of same people but different ages and clothing and hair styles
	Recognize same characters in picture books
Emotions	Cut, paste, match pictures of people with similar emotional expression
Assembling objects	Flashlight
	Battery-operated toys
	Model cars
	Screws and nuts
	Pens
Storing objects	Match grocery item to storage location
	Sort fruit and vegetables
	Sort different types of cereal

Form 7.9. Blank data form for natural and experience-based teaching of matching and sorting skills.

Data Form for Natural and Experience

Child _____   Teacher _____

Skill Area Matching and Sorting _____

Target Skill	Task Setup		Consequence
	Material or Task	Instruction	

EXAMPLE TASKS: VISUAL LEARNING

Example Task I: Matching and Sorting Similar Objects

- The child takes the *working* picture off her or his activity schedule, which shows a sequence of daily activities, such as singing, working, using the computer, eating a snack, and playing on the playground.
- The child brings the picture to the work area and places it on a vacant Velcro slot next to another picture of *working*.
- On the table, a plastic or cardboard strip indicates through the number of Velcro patches how many tasks the child has to do (the *work* card).
- Underneath all work slots an empty Velcro with a smiley face shows what happens once the child has finished his or her work.
- The child selects the picture of a liked object or activity and places it on this slot.
- Matching and sorting tasks are found on the left side of the table in separate drawers of a storage cart or underneath each other on a shelf.
- On the right side, a "finish" box indicates where the child is to put completed items.
- The child takes a tray labeled with the number *I* from the shelf. On this tray there is a smaller one to the left with unsorted forks, knives, and big and small spoons. To the right is a sorting tray with four compartments.
- Once the child has sorted the entire tray of cutlery, she or he sticks the number *I* on the work card and places the tray in the finish box.
- If the child makes a mistake, the therapist, who stands behind the child at a short distance, corrects him or her without any comment.
- The child then takes tray number 2 from the shelf and completes it.
- The child takes a third tray and, once he or she has completed all tasks, he or she places the working picture in a small finish box.

Prerequisites
The child is able to:
- sort cutlery and other tasks on his or her cart or shelf
- follow pictured activity schedules independently
- work from left to right
- place completed tasks into the finish box
- place completed picture instructions in the correct location
- recognize that work leads to reinforcement

Variations
- Instead of being labeled with numbers, tasks can be labeled with symbols, words, pictures, or photos that are used as instructions on the Velcro strip as well as on the trays.
- Various matching and sorting activities can be attempted, such as matching objects to pictures and matching pictures to pictures, letters, numbers, amounts, or words.
- Tasks such as cooking and baking, filing (e.g., stapling, hole-punching), assembling (e.g., model cars, screws and nuts), and measuring can also be arranged in a left-to-right format to suggest a sequence of necessary steps.

Note
The above procedure is characteristic of TEACCH methods (http://www.teacch.com) for developing sorting and matching skills and independence.

Task Example 2: Assembling Objects

- ShoeboxTasks are a line of products that facilitate independent matching, sorting, and assembling for young children, adolescents, and adults with ASD (see Figure 7.7).

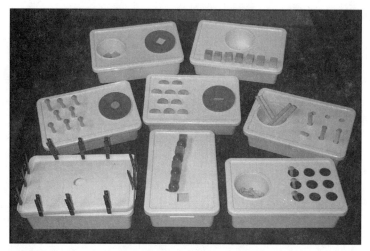

FIGURE 7.7. ShoeboxTasks help children become independent in skills such as matching, sorting, and assembling. (Source: www.shoeboxtasks.com)

- The child is cued by pictures on how to assemble nuts and bolts and how to package them.
- The therapist asks the child to "Do your work," supporting the verbal instruction with the picture or hand sign for *work*.
- The therapist stands in the background, providing support only when needed.
- Once the task is successfully completed, it is placed in the finish box.
- After the completion of all tasks the child is praised. She or he can exchange the picture of a re-inforcer for the actual item or activity.

Variation
In the beginning, one (then later three to five) ShoeboxTask is placed in front of the child.

Form 7.10 shows how these examples could be recorded using the blank data form for visual learning in Appendix 7.B.

Form 7.10. Example data form for visual learning method of teaching matching and sorting skills.

Data Form for Visual Lear

Child _____   Teacher _____

Skill Area Matching and Sorting

Target Skill	Task	Instruction	
		Verbal	Visual
Identical objects	Cutlery	"Match"	Picture of sorted cutlery
Assembling objects	Screws and nuts	"Do your work"	Pictures of assemble material

Related Literature

More information on ShoeboxTasks by Ron Larsen can be found at http://www.shoe
boxtasks.com.

Boswell, S. (2005). *TEACCH preschool curriculum guide.* Chapel Hill, NC: Division
TEACCH, University of North Carolina at Chapel Hill.

Boswell, S., Reynolds, B., Faulkner, R., & Benson, M. (2006). *Let's get started!* Chapel Hill,
NC: Division TEACCH, University of North Carolina at Chapel Hill.

Earles-Vollrath, T., Cook, K. T., & Ganz, J. B. (2006). *How to develop and implement visual
supports.* Austin, TX: PRO-ED.

Eckenrode, L., Fennell, P., & Hearsay, K. (2003, 2004). *Tasks galore.* Raleigh, NC: Tasks
Galore.

Schopler, E., Reichler, R. J., Bashford, A., Lansing, M. D., & Marcus, L. M. (1990). *The
Psychoeducational Profile–Revised.* Austin, TX: PRO-ED.

Section Overview

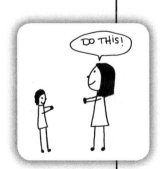

IMPORTANCE OF IMITATION

Imitation is an important step in the development of cognitive, communicative, and social skills. By imitating motor movements, sounds, gestures, facial expressions, and postures, children learn to understand contingencies and to develop communication, social behavior, play, and independence. They also learn about cause and effect when they realize that their sounds, movements, postures, and actions affect others. For example, crying may lead to getting the milk one wants, and turning the head signals that one has eaten enough (Piaget, 1962). Eye contact, speech, nonverbal communication, and the expression of emotions are crucially influenced by imitation skills. The acquisition of social rules, play skills, and even simple self-help skills like brushing teeth would be very difficult without the ability to imitate.

Why is imitation important?

- Understanding contingencies
- Forming the foundation of communication
- Referencing the interaction partner
- Learning social rules
- Learning to play
- Learning self-help skills

At the tender age of 1 year, nonautistic infants already are able to imitate simple gestures like saying "Bye" and to pretend they are drinking from an empty cup. By age 2 years, children are able to imitate two-step sequences and actions they have seen, even after some time has passed (Quill, 2002).

Many autistic children, however, have problems imitating actions (Sigman & Ungerer, 1984). Studies have shown that while children with ASD are considerably superior to children with Down syndrome in tasks of visual differentiation, such as the classification of pictures, letters, and word cards, they have comparatively fewer skills in imitating movements and gestures (Bernard-Opitz, 1983). To boost the imitation skills of these children, tasks for this manual have been selected that are fun, are functional, and serve a communicative purpose.

KEY QUESTIONS FOR EVALUATING A CHILD'S SKILLS

Observations of children with ASD can lead to the creation of motivating imitation exercises, adjusted to the individual's best learning channels (see list below). While some children benefit from the mass trials of the discrete trial format, others show better attention during a fast succession of imitation exercises offered by precision teaching. Yet others can be motivated best to imitate in front of a mirror, at a computer, in the sandbox, in a play group, in a singing group, or in the swimming pool, which would be common methods in natural and experience-based training.

Questions that help determine the best way for a child to learn

- Does the child imitate better with sensory materials (e.g., toys that spin, switches, lights)?
- Does the child imitate better when he or she sees himself or herself (e.g., in the mirror, as a shadow)?
- Does the child imitate better when music is involved (e.g., musical instruments, language songs, aerobics)?
- Does the child imitate better when he or she feels something (e.g., water, sand, lather)?
- Does the child imitate better with objects that resemble his or her self-stimulations or interests?
- Does the child imitate better with children of his or her same age?
- Does the child imitate better when he or she receives positive reinforcement (e.g., when he or she is thrown in the air for the imitation of "Raise your arms!")?
- Does the child imitate better in structured situations, at a table, or in play situations?
- Does the child imitate better when sequences of movement are fast or slow?

Tom, 4 years old, refused to participate in imitation exercises. When we noticed that he loved to be thrown in the air, we rewarded him with this whenever he imitated our gesture of arms stretching up. He learned within a few trials that his arm stretching led to the favorite game. A short time later he learned the mouth position of *u* and later the whole word "up."

Tanja, 5 years old, had a hard time learning the hand sign for *chip* (brushing her thumb under her chin). At a home visit I noted that she imitated various movements much faster in front of the mirror. In this setting, imitation of the *chip* hand sign posed no problem.

John, 4 years old, was highly unmotivated to imitate hand clapping. However, when various movements such as touching head, patting table, or stamping feet were requested in rapid sequence, he "woke up" and participated enthusiastically.

DEVELOPMENTAL LEVELS FOR IMITATION

At the age of 12 months, a typically developing infant is able to imitate simple movements such as waving, making simple sounds, and saying first words such as "Mama," "ball," or "bye-bye." At the age of 18 to 20 months, the toddler is able to imitate two-word sequences (Harris & Liebert, 1987; Kiphard, 1996). At this age, the child can imitate even several hours after observing the original model. Behavior the toddler has never seen before, such as sweeping the floor or painting one's lips, is modeled without prior practice.

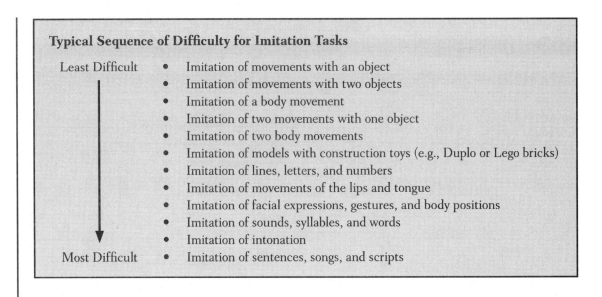

The sequence of difficulty for imitation tasks shows a wide spectrum. For some children, imitating static models such as pictures, written text, or built models is much easier than imitating dynamic models such as body movement, sounds, words, or sentences. Because dynamic models disappear right after their presentation, a child must possess good visual memory to imitate them. Imitations that make use of an object are usually easier for children to do than imitations of motor movements. My colleagues and I have observed, for example, that bursting bubbles in the air with the palms of both hands is learned faster than simply clapping hands.

A computer program called Speech Viewer has been helpful in developing vocal imitation in children with ASD. If the child makes a sound, pictures on the computer screen, such as balloons or the movement of a climbing monkey, change. One study demonstrated that children imitate more sounds during a period spent on the computer than a time of play interaction with their mothers and therapists using similar play material (Bernard-Opitz, Sriram, & Sapuan, 1999). Children with monotonous speech tone or a singsong voice can benefit from imitating different voices and speech tones. In addition to computer programs, many children find role-play speaking in the voice of different characters motivating.

HOW TO CONDUCT THE TRAINING

Within the **discrete trial format,** imitations of movements with objects are usually done with the therapist sitting opposite the child. A table or serving tray between child and therapist commonly holds the objects. At the beginning of training, an object such as a call bell is placed on the child's side and an identical one is placed on the therapist's side. The therapist presses his bell and requests the child to "do the same." If the child imitates within 3 seconds, she is reinforced. Once at least 80% of the imitations are successful on 2 consecutive days, the therapist begins the next teaching step—to discriminate two movements with two objects. In this step, the therapist may activate his bell three times before starting a new imitation, such as shaking a rattle three times.

Once imitation with objects is mastered, the child can begin learning imitations with movements, such as walking one's fingers on the table, clapping hands, changing oral–motor positions, or even making sounds. At a later therapy stage increasingly difficult imitations can be offered, such as imitating drawing or writing movements, built models, words, sentences, speech intonation, body positions, or gestures.

Once simple imitations are mastered, automatic production can be facilitated using **precision teaching.** Here, the frequency of imitation or copying is increased to allow fluid responding. Is the child able to imitate 35 to 50 movements in 1 minute? Can she or he copy that many letters in 1 minute?

For therapists using **natural and experience-based instruction,** imitation training is conducted in daily living and play settings that interest the child. Does the child imitate activities such as throwing, rolling, kicking, or tapping during ball play?

In **visual learning** programs, such as TEACCH, children copy specific models ranging from block designs to Lego-built cars, or they follow complex baking recipes.

TRAINING PROGRAM OVERVIEW

Form 7.11 outlines training programs to develop imitation skills. The listed teaching targets should be assessed prior to the intervention and following a period of training. Once the child's profile of skills, learning channels, and interests has been determined, the therapist can select one of the four subsequent teaching methods. A reproducible copy of the form can be found in Appendix 7.A.

Form 7.11. Overview of the STEP training programs for imitation skills; can be used as a pretest and posttest.

STEP Training Overview:
Imitation

Child _____ Teacher _____

❏ Pretest   ❏ Posttest

Imitation Skill	Task	Date Tested	Child's Response +	Child's Response −	Notes
Movements with an object	Place marble in bucket Use noisemaker Put on cap, sunglasses Move a toy car, animal, puppet				
Sequences of movement with two objects	First use a hammer, then move a car First comb hair, then blow nose First spray window, then spray a mirror				
A body movement	Clap hands Raise arms Nod				
Sequences of body movements	First touch head, then touch belly First crawl, then run				
Built and pictured models	Create blocks model Create Duplo and Lego model				

EXAMPLES OF DISCRETE TRIAL FORMAT

Example Task 1: Imitation of Placing Objects, Balls, or Coins Into a Bucket or Can

- Child and therapist sit facing each other (see Figure 7.8).
- The therapist holds a small bucket between his or her knees.
- The therapist has a variety of plastic balls next to his or her chair.
- The therapist holds up a plastic ball at the child's eye level, alerting the child to it.
- Once the child looks at the object and the therapist, the therapist throws the ball into the bucket.
- The therapist gives the child a ball with the request, "Put it in!"
- If the child throws the ball into the bucket, he or she is immediately praised and reinforced.
- If the child does not respond or throws the ball away, the therapist guides him or her so that together they throw the ball into the bucket.
- The exercise is repeated about 10 times.

Variation
Other objects, such as Lego bricks, cars, or coins, can be used instead of balls.

Example Task 2: Imitation of Sounds, Syllables, and Words

- Child and therapist sit facing each other.
- The therapist models a simple vowel, such as *aaa, ooo, uuu,* or *eee,* stressing clear mouth positions.
- If needed, the therapist prompts mouth positions by gently tapping the child's chin for *aaa,* touching the corner of the mouth for *eee,* or shaping the lips for *ooo* and *uuu.*
- In the beginning, the child is reinforced for successive approximations of the target behavior such as opening his or her mouth after hearing the model sound and making any sound within 3 seconds of the model.

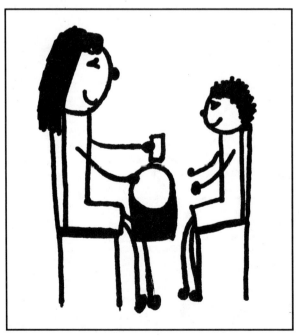

FIGURE 7.8. In the beginning of imitation training, the child learns that correct imitations, such as throwing something into a bucket, are reinforced.

- At a later stage, only the accurate reproduction of the sound modeled is reinforced.
- The exercise is repeated about 10 times.

Variations
- After successful imitation of one sound, a new sound is introduced.
- At the next stage, the mastered sounds are discriminated in blocks of five, then three, and, later, in random order (e.g., for five trials the therapist models *aaa*, followed by five trials of modeling *eee*).
- The imitation of more difficult sounds is practiced at a later stage.

Note
Sound combinations that are either in the child's repertoire or part of motivating objects or actions are more likely to be imitated.

Form 7.12 shows how these examples could be recorded using the blank data form for discrete trial format in Appendix 7.B.

Related Literature

Leaf, R., & McEachin, J. (1999). *A work in progress.* New York: DRL Books.

Maurice, C., Green, G., & Luce, S. L. (1996). *Behavioral intervention for young children with autism.* Austin, TX: PRO-ED.

EXAMPLES FOR PRECISION TEACHING

Example Task 1: Imitation of Movements with Objects

- The child and therapist stand facing each other and roll, throw, bounce, or kick the ball to each other.

Form 7.12. Example data form for discrete trial format method of teaching imitation skills.

Data Form for Discrete Trial

Child _____   Teacher _____

Skill Area __Imitation_____

In addition to recording the child's performance, indicate specifics about the task setup, s
schedule. Try to conduct about 10 trials per date and five sessions per week. Note that if the
Plot data on daily learning graphs.

Target Skill	Task Setup		Prompt	Consequence
	Material or Task	Instruction		
Movements with an object	Balls; bucket	"Put it in"	Physical guidance	Verbal and material reinforcement
Sounds, syllables, words, speech, melody		"Say aaa (or ooo or uuu or eee)"	Mouth position	Verbal and material reinforcement

- As the therapist rolls the ball to the child, he or she says, "Roll the ball."
- The child is praised for rolling the ball back.
- The therapist sets the timer for 20 seconds and counts out loud or otherwise keeps track of the number of successful imitations.
- The therapist shows the result to the child.
- The child receives a token when he or she exceeds his or her previous imitation rate.
- When the child has improved his or her performance three times or has reached his or her final performance aim, he or she receives a reinforcer.
- Over the course of the session, the rate of ball playing is successively increased.

Variation

Modeling of different play activities is done in blocks of five or three, or in random order.

Cross-Reference

Depending on the individual child, receptive and expressive language can be trained during this task. For example, for receptive language, the therapist would say, "Roll the ball" (hear–do). For expressive language, the therapist would say, "We roll the ball; say 'Roll the ball'" (hear–say). Or, the therapist would say, "What does the ball do?" and wait for the child's response (see–say).

Task Example 2: Imitation of Sequence of Movements with Two Objects—Squirt with a Squirt Bottle

- The child and therapist face a mirror in a bathroom.
- The therapist demonstrates with a squirt bottle or water pistol how to squirt water onto the mirror, the window, or the shower walls.
- The therapist hands the child a second bottle and instructs, "Do this."
- The child is praised for imitation.
- The therapist sets the timer for 20 seconds and counts aloud or otherwise tracks the number of squirts to the modeled locations.
- The child receives a token when he or she exceeds his or her previous imitation rate.
- When the child has improved his or her performance three times or has reached his or her final performance aim, he or she receives a reinforcer.

Variation

The squirting task moves to different objects and locations, such as outside to squirt plants, trees, or the sidewalk.

Cross-Reference

- Besides teaching the imitation of movements, this exercise also strengthens finger and hand muscles, an important prerequisite for drawing and writing. To strengthen the pincer grasp (thumb and forefinger only), the child can squeeze squeaky toys or the pumps of small medicine bottles.
- Other movements involved in drawing and writing, such as flexing the wrist or repeatedly making the "okay" sign, can also be modeled following the above procedure of squeezing squeaky toys or bottle pumps.

Task Example 3: Imitation of Sequences of Body Movement

- Child and therapist sit or stand facing each other.
- The therapist sets the timer for 20 seconds.
- The therapist positions himself or herself to the child's eye level and tries to catch his or her attention.
- He or she instructs, "Do this," modeling movements such as clapping, stomping, or putting the hands on the head or the finger on the nose.
- When the timer rings, the therapist records the child's performance and provides a token when the performance level increases.

- When the child has improved his or her performance three times or has reached his or her final performance aim, he or she receives a reinforcer.
- This task is illustrated in Figure 7.9.

Task Example 4: Copying Strokes, Letters, or Numbers

- The therapist passes the child a piece of lined paper with a sequence of three strokes on it in different directions. They can be components of letters or numbers.
- The therapist instructs, "Copy the pattern as fast as you can and as many times as you can."
- The therapist counts well-done strokes or asks the child to self-check.
- The number of strokes made in 20 seconds is noted.
- When the child has improved his or her performance three times or has reached his or her final performance aim, he or she receives a reinforcer.

Note

"See–do" tasks usually can be done with 35 to 60 correct responses per minute. Individual speed should be considered, though, when setting fluency aims.

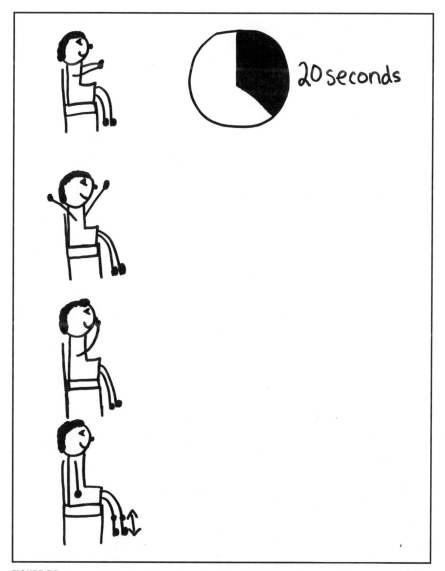

FIGURE 7.9. In precision teaching, time limits help children learn to imitate movements increasingly more fluently.

Form 7.13. Example data form for precision teaching of imitation skills.

Target Skill	Task Setup		Time Unit	Consequence	Le... Hi...
	Material or Task	**Instruction**			
Movements with an object	Throw, roll, or bounce ball	"Roll the ball"	20 seconds	Praise and smiley	Se...
Sequences of movements with two objects	Squirt on mirror and window	"Do this"	20 seconds	Praise and smiley	Se...
Sequences of body movement	Make fast movements, such as clapping hands and st...	"Do this"	20 seconds	Praise and smiley	Se...

(Form header: Data Form for Precision Te... / Child ___ / Teacher ___ / Skill Area __Imitation__)

Form 7.13 shows how these examples could be recorded using the blank data form for precision teaching in Appendix 7.B.

EXAMPLES FOR NATURAL AND EXPERIENCE-BASED TEACHING

Example Task 1: Imitation of Movements with Objects

- The child and the therapist have two small balls of dough each and a rolling pin and a cookie cutter between them.
- The therapist holds his dough ball and the rolling pin at eye level and says, "Watch!"
- Once the child attends, the therapist rolls the dough and presses the cutter into the dough.
- Once the child has imitated the model successfully, the therapist praises the child.
- Functional reinforcers are used. For example, after imitating the cookie cutting, the child can be allowed to eat a baked cookie.

Variations

- The child can attempt several activities with the dough: pounding, stamping, and scratching patterns.
- The child imitates bead stringing, then is allowed to wear the bead necklace.
- The child imitates building a tower, then can knock it over.
- The child imitates cut-and-paste activities, noisemakers, or musical instruments in one-to-one or group activities.

Example Task 2: Imitation of Body Movements

- The child and therapist stand facing each other.
- The therapist tries to get the child's attention.

- The therapist stretches his hands up high and says, "Up" or "Do this!"
- If the child imitates the movement, the therapist praises the child and lifts him or her in the air, saying, "Up." See Figure 7.10.
- If the child does not react or reacts incorrectly, the therapist guides his or her arms to the correct position.
- Prompted trials are praised, but not reinforced with the natural reinforcer.
- The game is repeated as often as the child likes, up to 15 times.

Variations

- The child attempts imitation of other body movements, such as stretching arms to the side to "fly" around the therapist, stretching arms to the front to request swinging through the legs of the therapist, and rolling hands over each other to request to do a somersault.
- The child makes yes, *no*, or *please* gestures to request liked objects or activities, or reject disliked objects or activities.
- Imitation exercises can involve several children.
- The child can practice music, songs, or aerobic movements in front of a mirror or as shadow games.

Table 7.3 provides examples of how natural teaching can be used to develop imitation skills. Form 7.14 shows a data form that can be used to record a child's responses to natural teaching. This form can be reproduced from Appendix 7.B.

Related Literature

Quill, K. A. (2002). *Do, watch, listen, say.* Baltimore: Brookes.

Bondy, A., Dickey, D., & Buswell, S. (2002). *The pyramid approach to education: Lesson plans for young children.* Newark, DE: Pyramid Educational Products.

EXAMPLES FOR VISUAL LEARNING

Example Task I: Imitation of Movements with One Object

- The therapist and child sit facing each other. To the left of the child a tray contains pairs of noise-makers (e.g., two drums, two bells, two rattles).

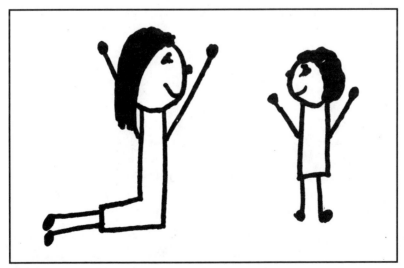

FIGURE 7.10. Once the child imitates lifting his or her arms, the therapist lifts the child in the air.

Table 7.3
Examples of Ways Natural and Experience-Based Teaching
Can Be Used To Develop Imitation Skills

Imitation Skill	Examples
Movements with an object	Toys • Push car, rock baby doll • Pop bubbles in the air or on the table • Squash shaving foam Sound Activities • Use noisemakers • Play musical instruments • Bang pot, lid • Ring bell, rattle Art activities • Imitate big and small movements when drawing or writing (horizontal, vertical, circle, triangle) • Roll, press, stamp, or cut dough or play-dough Everyday activities • Stir spoon in cup • Sharpen pencil • Open book • Pour juice • Put away or take objects • Comb hair • Brush teeth
Body movement	• Wave, nod or shake head • Make "good" or "okay" hand sign • Make gestures for eating, drinking, tired, up, down • Clap, stamp • Run, crawl, turn • Arms up, to the side, down
Facial expression, gestures, body positions	• Play "Simon says" • Play language songs with various movement patterns • Imitate animals, mime, gesture (e.g., shadow games, in front of mirror, with frozen TV screen)
Sounds, syllables, words, scripts	• Say sound chains • Interrupt songs • Say, "Ready, steady, go!"

- The therapist directs the child's attention to one of the noisemakers (e.g., the drum) while activating it. He or she passes the corresponding second object (e.g., the other drum) to the child and instructs, "Do this."
- The therapist reinforces appropriate imitating and places the pair of noisemakers into the finish box. See Figure 7.11.
- The next pair of noisemakers is then used.

Variations
- To enhance attention, pairs of noisemakers are taken from a feely bag or a closed box.
- After the therapist models, the child is instructed to activate various objects that have sensory properties similar to his or her self-stimulations (e.g., spinning tops).

Form 7.14. Blank data form for natural and experience-based teaching of imitation skills.

Data Form for Natural and Experienc

Child _____ Teacher _____

Skill Area ___Imitation_____

Target Skill	Task Setup		Consequence
	Material or Task	**Instruction**	

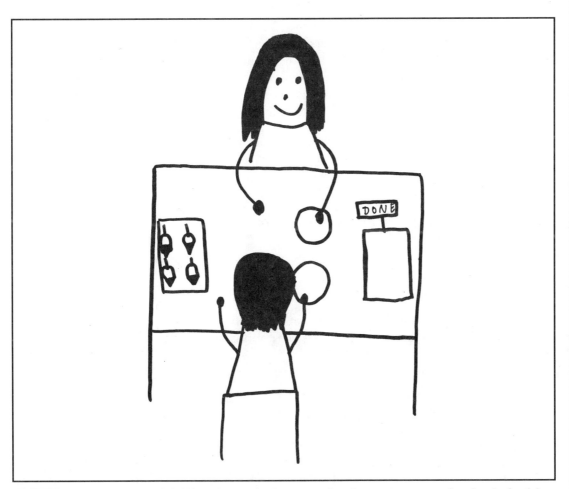

FIGURE 7.11. Once therapist and child have beaten the drums together, the instruments are placed in the finish box.

Example Task 2: Imitation of Body Movements

- The child and therapist sit facing each other.
- The therapist offers the child a liked activity, such as stringing beads, building a tower, blowing bubbles, pushing a car down a ramp, eating food, or drinking a beverage.
- Before allowing the child to take another bead, block, or other item, he or she is requested, through picture card, word card, or hand sign, to imitate a simple activity such as clapping hands, stomping feet, or nodding head.
- Once the child has imitated successfully, he is allowed the next bead, block, or other item.

Variations

- The child imitates knocking (e.g., on the table, at the door, at the window).
- The child imitates songs, puppet play.
- The child imitates in a small group (e.g., "Simon says: All children crawl ...").
- The child imitates sequences (e.g., first clapping hands, then stamping feet).

Example Task 3: Imitation of Built or Drawn Models

- The child takes the picture of *working* from a pictured activity sequence.
- The child brings it to the work table and attaches it to a Velcro strip that contains a sequence of the numbers 1, 2, and 3.
- The child takes a tray numbered *1* from a shelf. The tray contains blocks and a pictured building model.
- Once the child has built the pictured model, he or she puts the completed tray into the finish box.
- The child attaches number *1* from his or her Velcro strip to the number *1* on the shelf and retrieves tray number 2.
- If the child makes a mistake in any part of the task, the therapist corrects silently.
- Once the child has mastered all tasks, she or he puts the *working* picture in a corresponding *done* slot at the end of the above-mentioned pictured schedule.

Prerequisites

- The child has mastered the requested activity.
- The child can complete pictured sequences independently.
- The child knows that completed tasks are placed in the finish box.
- The child knows that completed pictured instructions are put into the done slot.

Variations

- Instead of using numbers, the therapist can attach pictures or words representing the tasks to Velcro strips.
- Various sorting, matching, and independent work tasks can be completed according to the above method.

Notes

- Figure 7.12 shows an example of a model that can be assembled using a picture sequence.
- TEACCH training workshops and Web sites with materials and tasks provide more detailed information on this method.

Form 7.15 shows how these examples could be recorded using the blank data form for visual teaching in Appendix 7.B.

Related Literature

Frost, L., & Bondy, A. (2002). *The Picture Exchange Communication System.* Newark, DE: Pyramid Educational Products.

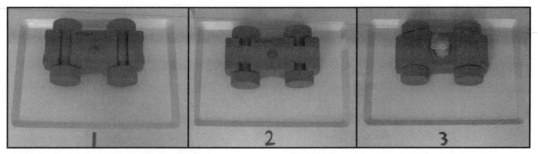

FIGURE 7.12. A model, such as this car, can be independently constructed using a sequence of pictures showing necessary construction steps.

Form 7.15. Example data form for visual learning method of teaching imitation skills.

Data Form for Visual Lear

Child _____   Teacher _____

Skill Area __Imitation_____

Target Skill	Task	Instruction	
		Verbal	**Visual**
Movements with an object	Noisemakers	"Do this"	Pairs of noisemakers; picture or hand sign for "Do this"
A body movement	Clap hands, lift arms, or nod head	"Do this"	Picture or hand sign for "Do this"
Built and pictured models		"Build this" or "Draw this"	Built or drawn mode

Schopler, E., Lansing, M., & Waters, L. (1983). *Individualized assessment and treatment for autistic and developmentally disabled children.* Baltimore: University Park Press.

Quill, K. A. (2002). *Do, watch, listen, say.* Baltimore: Brookes.

For more information on Tasks Galore, see http://www.tasksgalore.com

For more information on TEACCH, see http://www.teacch.com

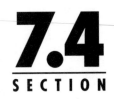
Section Overview

Importance of Language Comprehension

Key Questions for Evaluating a Child's Skills

Developmental Levels for Language Comprehension

How To Conduct the Training

Training Program Overview

Examples of Discrete Trial Format

Examples of Precision Teaching

Examples for Experience-Based Teaching

Examples for Visual Teaching

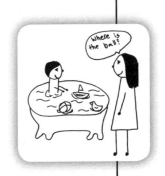

IMPORTANCE OF LANGUAGE COMPREHENSION

Language comprehension is a key prerequisite of social and communicative behavior. Children need to be able to follow instructions and understand names of objects, people, and events. They need to know words that denote action and description, as well as location, time, and sequence. Children first learn to respond to simple instructions and, in general, progress through to the understanding of more complex instructions. For children to be integrated into preschool, kindergarten, and first grade, it is often as important to be able to comprehend language and adapt to social rules as it is to have mastered the basic steps of toilet training. As early as kindergarten, children are expected to follow instructions such as, "Come here," "Sit down," "Go to the toilet," "Take the red crayon," and "Now we all go swimming." Children who do not listen or do not consistently respond to instructions are often alienated from regular settings.

Why train language comprehension?

- Understanding instructions
- Controlling behavior
- Enhancing active language
- Improving attention
- Improving auditory differentiation
- Facilitating abstract thinking
- Developing basic preacademic skills
- Understanding rules

Most children with ASD have to be specifically taught nouns and verbs and concepts such as color, shape, size, opposites, numbers, and letters. Comprehension facilitates expression. As their language comprehension increases, children tend to use more frequent and more differentiated active speech.

According to the staff of a group home, 8-year-old Susan understood "everything." To demonstrate Susan's level of comprehension, her instructor gestured toward the toilet and instructed Susan to sit, which she immediately did. Susan also pulled up her pants after toileting and followed the command to flush the toilet. The instructor was taken by surprise, however, when the girl completed the behavioral chain and washed her hands upon my completely unrelated command: "The chickens have to be fed." Obviously Susan had compensated for her lack of comprehension by reacting to visual signals and by memorizing activity chains.

Parents may not realize that their children do not comprehend everything they say. Training programs that offer systematic steps in developing language comprehension, therefore, can be extremely beneficial.

The occupational therapist instructed Jeanne to get the "big spoon" from the kitchen. When the girl returned with the small spoon, the therapist sent Jeanne back, stressing that she should get the "BIG spoon." A short time later, Jeanne brought the big fork. The therapist, meanwhile, was obviously unnerved and repeated herself: "I said the BIG SPOON." After another two erroneous attempts, child and therapist were at their wits' end. Jeanne cried and bit her hand, and once she had calmed down we gave her the choice of a big and a small spoon. It became obvious that Jeanne had not yet mastered this discrimination.

This example illustrates that behavior problems can sometimes be caused by deficits in comprehension and should not be interpreted as intentionally oppositional behavior.

KEY QUESTIONS FOR EVALUATING A CHILD'S SKILLS

Interviews with parents and observation of the child in everyday settings are helpful ways of getting a first impression of the child's skill at differentiating sounds and understanding language. Developing a profile of the child's strengths and deficits, as well as his or her learning channels, interests, and motivation levels, forms the basis for interventions.

Questions that help determine the best way for a child to learn

Does the child:

- react to loud sounds?
- notice environmental sounds, such as sirens, thunder, a barking dog, a slamming door?
- follow instructions, such as "Stop," "Wait," "Come here," and "Sit down"?
- respond to instructions to bring familiar objects to named people, such as, "Give the key to Mom"?
- react to speech without visual cues?
- comprehend instructions better when they are paired with gestures, eye pointing, or situational cues?
- attend to symbols, pictures, or written words?
- discriminate different instructions, such as, "Give," "Take," "Eat," "Play"?
- respond to complex instructions, such as, "Do your homework first and then you can watch TV for 15 minutes"?
- understand instructions with several components, such as when the teacher says, "Tomorrow morning we will meet at the gym at 8:30 A.M."?

DEVELOPMENTAL LEVELS FOR LANGUAGE COMPREHENSION

During the first half-year of life, typically developing infants are able to turn their head to a sound source and look at the speaker. At about 1 year of age, they look at the person named, react to "No," and make gestures such as waving "Bye-bye" on request. At age 18 months, they can label most common objects and about four body parts. At the age of 2 years, their language comprehension includes about 20 objects and 15 pictures, and they can understand questions with two alternatives. At 3 to 3-and-a-half years, they point to pictures denoting actions, colors, shapes, and simple comparisons (e.g., bigger vs. smaller; Brigance, 2004; Johnson-Martin et al., 1990; Kiphard, 1996).

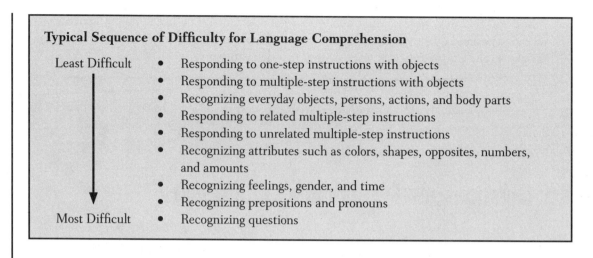

The above levels of difficulty show the normal sequence of language comprehension development integrated with a logical analysis of task levels. The sequence and selection of the tasks presented in this section, which are fun and meaningful, is based on the knowledge that motivation is crucial for children with ASD to learn.

Parents of infants with ASD often notice early on that their children do not react to common environmental sounds. Their infants may, however, respond to certain sounds they find interesting, such as the rustling of chocolate paper—or, as was the case of an adolescent with ASD, the sound of onions being peeled from the room next door. Frequently, children with ASD do not respond to simple instructions and only exhibit situational language comprehension. For instance, they understand that the milk goes into the refrigerator because Mom is pointing in that direction and they can remember that it belongs there.

How To Conduct the Training

Tasks for language comprehension can be conducted at a table, during play, while out walking, or in any other setting. For children with minimal understanding, structured sessions are usually a good starting point. One of the standard tasks to facilitate basic compliance can be conducted using the discrete trial format. The therapist sits facing the child at a distance of about 6 feet. The child is instructed to approach the adult on the command and gesture of "Come here." Upon reaching the adult, the child is reinforced by praise, a hug, tickles, a small food item, or another previously identified reinforcing consequence. The task is repeated about 10 times. Once the child has mastered the behavior, a new command can be taught. (Mastery is assumed when the child has made 80% or more correct responses on two occasions or 100% correct responses on one occasion.) To test the child's ability to discriminate, mastered responses can be mixed with other known commands, such as, "Sit down," "Throw the paper in the trash can," and so forth. This ensures that the child is responding to the command itself and not just to the sequence of being called and coming.

Some children are more motivated in less structured settings. When walking in the park, they can be taught to interrupt their walking, running, or skipping upon the command of "Stop." This game can be made more advanced, where the therapist instructs the children to "Walk," "Crawl," "Skip," or "Walk backwards" (see Figure 7.13). Even two-step commands can be taught in a playful manner, such as, "Turn around and jump." With peers or siblings as models, this can be a motivating game.

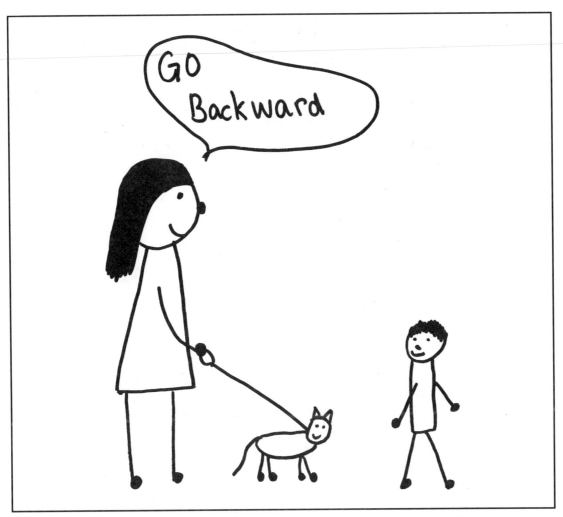

FIGURE 7.13. Even during a walk, parents and others can improve the child's language comprehension.

After the child understands about five basic instructions, comprehension of people and objects can be taught: "Pass this to Mom," or "Put the ball away." Later, the comprehension of body parts, clothing items, locations, and concepts is taught. As with other skills, the selection of the training method depends on the child's level of skill, attention, and interest. Is the child more attentive when tasks are presented in a structured manner at a table (e.g., "Take the shoe"), during play (e.g., "Put the shoe on dolly"), in everyday settings (e.g., "Put your shoes on"), or when presented in the visual mode? Is the involvement of peer models helpful or distracting?

Some children learn to understand object labels faster with real objects, while others respond better to pictures, symbols, or word cards. The therapist should observe which tasks are learned faster with or without time limits. Fluency drills that require children to show a behavior quickly can help elicit automatic, spontaneous responding. When responses to commands such as, "Point to your hand/tummy/head/foot," or, at a more advanced level, "Point to 1:30 P.M./5:00 P.M./10:15 P.M.," are given at a fast rate, such as within a 20-second time period, generalization is more likely to occur. Because many children with ASD learn better when instructions are presented visually rather than in speech, therapists need to provide pictures, symbols, and written words when assessing optimal learning channels for comprehension. Regardless of the instructional methods, it is important to confirm that the child has generalized the mastered behavior to everyday settings.

TRAINING PROGRAM OVERVIEW

Form 7.16 outlines training programs to develop language comprehension skills. The listed teaching targets should be assessed prior to the intervention and following a period of training. Once the child's profile of skills, learning channels, and interests has been determined, the therapist can select one of the four subsequent teaching methods. A reproducible copy of the form can be found in Appendix 7.A.

EXAMPLES OF DISCRETE TRIAL FORMAT

Example Task 1: Responding to One-Step Instructions Without Objects

- The therapist sits facing the child at a distance of about 6 feet. An assistant stands behind the child.
- The child is instructed to approach the adult on the command and gesture (or picture) of "Come here."
- Upon reaching the adult, the child is reinforced by praise, a hug, tickles, a small food item, or another previously identified reinforcer.
- If the child fails to respond, the assistant physically guides him or her to the therapist, who reinforces the child.
- If the child tries to run away, the assistant prevents it and guides him or her back to the therapist's chair.
- The task is repeated 10 times.

Form 7.16. Overview of the STEP training programs for language comprehension; can be used as a pretest and posttest.

**STEP Training Overview:
Language Comprehension**

Child _____ Teacher _____

☐ Pretest   ☐ Posttest

Language Comprehension Skill	Task Examples	Date Tested	Child's Response +	Child's Response −	Notes
One-step instructions with objects	"Put in." "Ready, set, go." "One, two, and the last number is ... three!" "Eat the cookie." "Drink the juice."				
One-step instructions without objects	"Come here." "Sit down." "Stand up." "Wait." "Line up."				

Variations

- The distance between child and therapist is increased.
- Other people give the command.
- The seating arrangement and number of chairs are varied.
- The command is given in different settings (e.g., locations, seats, distances).
- The command is given from different positions (e.g., standing, walking). See Figure 7.14.

Notes

- After mastery of the first instruction ("Come here"), a second one is introduced ("Sit down").
- Once the child has mastered both instructions, the therapist teaches them as discriminations in blocks of five, blocks of three, and, finally, random sequence.
- The prompts (e.g., gestures or pictures, verbal stress) are faded with the child's progress.

Example Task 2: Comprehension of Emotions

- The child and therapist sit next to each other at a table.
- Four pictures with emotional expressions, such as happy, sad, angry, and frightened, are on the table.
- The therapist asks the child to "Point to the sad child."
- When the child responds correctly, he or she is praised and gets a token or a material reinforcer.
- When the child responds incorrectly, the instructor gives prompts, such as pointing to the correct picture or guiding the child's hand.
- Prompted tasks are reinforced by praise only.
- The task is repeated 10 times.

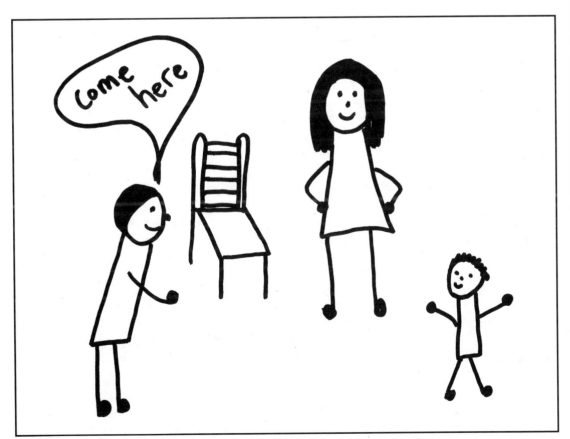

FIGURE 7.14. Both parents take turns instructing the child to come.

Variations

- The therapist exchanges cards that are mastered for new cards.
- The therapist can model the corresponding emotional expression and prompt the child to do the same.

Form 7.17 shows how these examples could be recorded using the blank data form for discrete trial format in Appendix 7.B.

Related Literature

Blank, M., McKirdy, L. S., & Payne, P. (2000). *Links to language.* Upper Montclair, NJ: HELP Associates.

Leaf, R., & McEachin, J. (1999). *A work in progress.* New York: DLR Books.

Lovaas, O. I. (1981). *Teaching developmentally disabled children: The me book.* Austin, TX: PRO-ED.

Maurice, C., Green, G., & Luce, S. L. (1996). *Behavioral intervention for young children with autism.* Austin, TX: PRO-ED.

EXAMPLES OF PRECISION TEACHING

Example Task I: Recognizing Pictures of Objects

- Therapist and child sit at the table.
- The child is asked to select a picture of something that he or she wants as a reward, such as some chips, a toy, or time on the computer.
- The reward picture is placed on a Velcro strip above three additional Velcro strips, which serve as cues for three tokens.

Form 7.17. Example data form for discrete trial format method of teaching language comprehension skills.

Data Form for Discrete Trial

Child _____ Teacher _____

Skill Area _Language Comprehension_____

In addition to recording the child's performance, indicate specifics about the task setup, schedule. Try to conduct about 10 trials per date and five sessions per week. Note that if the Plot data on daily learning graphs.

Target Skill	Task Setup		Prompt	Consequence
	Material or Task	**Instruction**		
One-step instructions with objects	Chair	"Come here." "Sit down."	Pointing; physical prompting	Praise; material or action reinforcer
Emotions	Pictures of various emotions	"Point to the sad child."	Pointing; physical prompting; distance prompt	Praise; material or action reinforcer

- The therapist puts six known pictures of everyday objects in a circle (see Figure 7.15).
- The therapist sets the timer for 20 seconds.
- In rapid sequence, the therapist asks the child to point to specific pictures ("Point to ball, Slinky, balloons").
- Correct responses are reinforced through nodding.
- When the child points to an incorrect picture, the therapist repeats the instruction and points to the correct picture.
- After 20 seconds the therapist writes down the number of correctly recognized pictures.
- If the child performs better than on the previous trial, he or she is allowed to put a Smiley on the token card.
- Once the child reaches three Smileys, she or he will receive the pictured reinforcer selected previously.

Variations
- The layout of the pictures (e.g., in a circle or square, horizontal, vertical) can be varied.
- Pictures with other teaching targets (e.g., verbs, adjectives, numbers) can be used.

Example Task 2: Discriminating Action Pictures

- The child and therapist sit opposite each other at a table with 10 everyday objects.
- For 20 seconds, the therapist instructs in steady succession: "Point to the sponge. Give me the cup. Take the book."
- Each correct response is counted and is reinforced by nodding.
- The child is prompted after incorrect responses, as in the previous example task.
- The numbers of correct and incorrect responses are recorded on a learning graph.
- The task is repeated until the child has reached his or her learning criteria or has improved the frequency of correct responses three times (see use of token card in previous task).

Variation
Actions such as clapping hands, walking, jumping, and skipping can also be requested within a short time period.

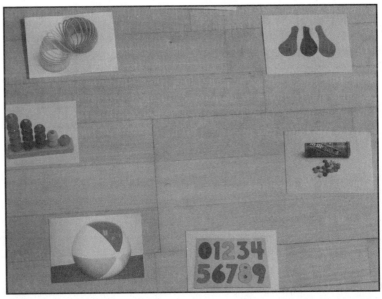

FIGURE 7.15. The child is asked to identify pictures quickly, such as, "Point to ball, Slinky, balloons."

Prerequisite

The child must be able to recognize the requested pictured objects and actions.

Example Task 3: Responding to Unrelated, Multiple-Step Instructions Involving Adjectives

- The child gets a page with 20 different shapes, colors, and sizes.
- The therapist sets the timer for 30 seconds.
- The therapist requests, "Point to the small, blue triangle." "Point to the big, yellow circle."
- The therapist records the number of items correctly recognized in a 30-second period.
- When the child improves his or her performance, he or she gets a token.
- The task is repeated until the child has reached his or her learning criteria or has improved the frequency of correct responses three times. The therapist can implement a token system of reinforcement where the child receives a token for each improvement in performance. Once the child has received a predetermined number of tokens (e.g., three), he or she exchanges them for a preferred item or activity.

Variations

- The layout of the pictures can be varied (e.g., circle, square, horizontal, vertical).
- The number of shapes and features the child must discriminate among can be increased with the child's progress.

Note

For this "Hear-Do" task, the therapist can expect 35 to 50 responses in 1 minute, although performance will vary among children.

Cross-Reference

The described task for language comprehension (Hear-Do) can be complemented by tasks for imitation (Hear-Say) and labeling (See-Say).

Form 7.18 shows how these examples could be recorded using the blank data form for precision teaching in Appendix 7.B.

Related Literature

Bondy, A., Dickey, D., & Buswell, S. (2002). *The pyramid approach to education: Lesson plans for young children*. Newark, DE: Pyramid Educational Products.

Partington, J. W., & Sundberg, M. L. (1998). *The assessment of basic language and learning skills*. Pleasant Hill, CA: Behavior Analysts.

EXAMPLES FOR EXPERIENCE-BASED TEACHING

Task Example 1: Responding to One-Step Instructions with Objects

- Therapist and child sit next to each other on the floor with two toy cars at a starting line.
- The therapist says slowly, "Ready, set ... go!" and lets her car go on the word "Go!" (see Figure 7.16).
- She repeats the instruction while looking at the child.
- If the child lets his or her car go upon the command, he or she is praised and is allowed to start the game again.

Form 7.18. Example data form for precision teaching of language comprehension skills.

Data Form for Precision Te

Child _____   Teacher _____

Skill Area _Language Comprehension_____

| Target Skill | Task Setup | | Time Unit | Consequence | Le: Hi |
	Material or Task	Instruction			
Objects	Ball	"Point to the ball."	Number of correct pictures identified in 20 seconds	Praise; token when performance is better than the previous trial	He
Discriminating actions	Sponge	"Point to the sponge."	Number of actions or object functions discriminated	Praise; token when performance is better than the previous trial	He
Adjectives	Pictures of shape	"Point to the small, blue	Number of correctly iden-	Praise; token when performance is	H

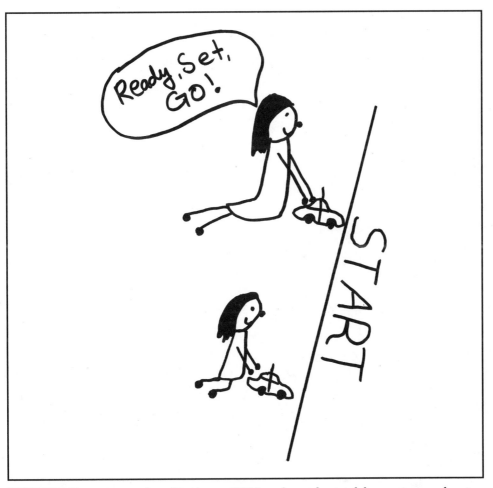

FIGURE 7.16. Play scripts, such as, "Ready, set, GO!," can be used to teach language comprehension.

- If he or she does not respond correctly, the therapist prompts the child.

Variations

- The task can be done with different play objects, such as a variety of cars (e.g., wind-up cars, pull-back cars), balls, marbles on a marble drop, blocks in a tower, or drums.
- This task can be expanded to a turn-taking activity. Upon instruction, therapist and child throw or roll balls to each other.
- The instruction can be changed to "One, two, and the last number is ... three!" The therapist can use other signal words, such as "soft" and "loud" for drumming, speaking, or singing softly and loudly.

Task Example 2: Recognizing Emotions

- The child and the therapist watch a videotape with real or cartoon people who show clear emotions.
- At a very specific emotionally laden scene, the therapist stops the tape and asks the child, "Who is scared?" "Show me the happy boy."
- If the child points correctly, the tape is forwarded to the next scene that has a clear emotion.
- If the child does not react, or identifies incorrectly, the therapist prompts by modeling or pointing to the correct emotional expression.

Note
Corresponding pictures or word cards can also prompt children with good visual skills.

Table 7.4 provides examples of how natural teaching can be used to develop language comprehension skills. Form 7.19 shows a data form that can be used to record a child's responses to natural teaching. This form can be reproduced from Appendix 7.B.

Form 7.19. Blank data form for natural and experience-based teaching of language comprehension skills.

Data Form for Natural and Experienc

Child _____ Teacher _____

Skill Area __Language Comprehension_____

Target Skill	Task Setup		Consequence
	Material or Task	**Instruction**	

Table 7.4
Examples of Ways Natural and Experience-Based Teaching Can Be Used To Develop Language Comprehension

Language Comprehension Skill	Setting/Activity	Example Instructions
One-step instructions with objects	Everyday settings	• "Open the door." "Turn on the light." "Put it in."
	Self-help	• "Eat the cookie." "Drink the juice." "Dry your hands." "Turn on the light." "Put the blocks (or dolls or tracks) back."
	Play	• "Color (or build or cut)." "Clean up." "Ready, steady, go!" "One, two, and the last number is … three."
One-step instructions without objects	Home	• "Come here." "Sit down." "Stand up." "Wait!" "Stop!" "Wave." "Say *hello* (or *bye*)."
	Kindergarten or school	• "Line up." "Get your snack." "Go play."
Objects	Play	• "Get the ball (or the doll or the Lego)."
	Self-help	• "Put on your shoes (or your jacket or your pants)."
People	Home	• "Daddy (or Mommy) has the cookie." "Where is your brother (or sister)?" "Pass the sugar to Aunt Mary."
	School	• "Bring the book to Mrs. Miller." "Borrow the scissors from Jana."
Actions and object functions	Play	• "Roll (or catch or tap or kick) the ball."
	Self-help	• "Put on your jacket." "Wash your hair."
	Play	• "Get something to build with."
	Self-help	• "What do you use for playing (or eating or wearing or driving)?"
Parts of the whole	Book	• "Point to the dog's tail." "Show me the wheels of the train."
Related multiple-step instructions	Play	• "Let the dog walk."
	Self-help	• "Get the scissors and cut."
Unrelated multiple-step instructions	"Simon Says" game	• "Go to the chair and turn around."
	Self-help	• "Get your jacket and turn off the light." • "Wash your face and your hands."
Categories	Play	• "Give the doll some vegetables."
	School	• "Draw some birds in the sky." "Color the fruits."
Sounds	Play	• "What do you hear?"
	Toy animals	• "What makes the sound *meow*?"
	Pairs of musical instruments (behind a partition)	• "Which instrument is this?" (bang, jingle, rattle)

(continues)

Table 7.4. *(Continued)*

Language Comprehension Skill	Setting/Activity	Example Instructions
Locations	Play with dollhouse	• "Put the Mommy (or Daddy) doll in the living room (or kitchen or bedroom)."
	Kindergarten or school	• "The bag of chips is on the sofa." • "Go to the playground (or the swing or the slide)." • "Bring this to the nurse's office."
Adjectives	Play	• "Get the red ball."
	Self-help	• "Put on the clean t-shirt." "Put on the long scarf." "Put it in the round box." "Take the big cookie." "Take two Smarties!"
	School	• "Draw four triangles."
Emotions	Magazine	• "Cut out the happy faces."
	Video	• "Show me who is scared (or happy or desperate)."
Gender	Play	• "Sit with the boys."
Singular and plural	Play	• "Get a ball (or the balls)."
	Self-help	• "Eat one (or many) grapes."
Prepositions	Play	• "The game is next to the shelf."
Pronouns	Self-help	• "The candies are in my bag."
Questions	Play	• "Who wants bubbles?"
	Self-help	• "Which ice cream do you want?"

EXAMPLES FOR VISUAL TEACHING

Task Example 1: Responding to Unrelated Multiple-Step Instructions

- A Velcro strip with 10 lined-up pictures (see Figure 7.17 for examples of pictures) and written instructions (often called a *mini-plan*) is placed in front of the child. The pictures and instructions show objects and actions involved in making a sandwich:

  — "Get the plate." "Get the knife." "Get the bread." "Get the Nutella."
  — "Put a slice of bread on your plate."
  — "Open the lid of the Nutella jar."
  — "Get the Nutella from the jar with your knife." "Spread it on your bread."
  — "Cut the bread in half."
  — "Eat the sandwich."

- If the child follows the pictured sequence, he or she is allowed to eat the sandwich.
- If he or she makes mistakes, the therapist, who is observing from behind, corrects them silently.

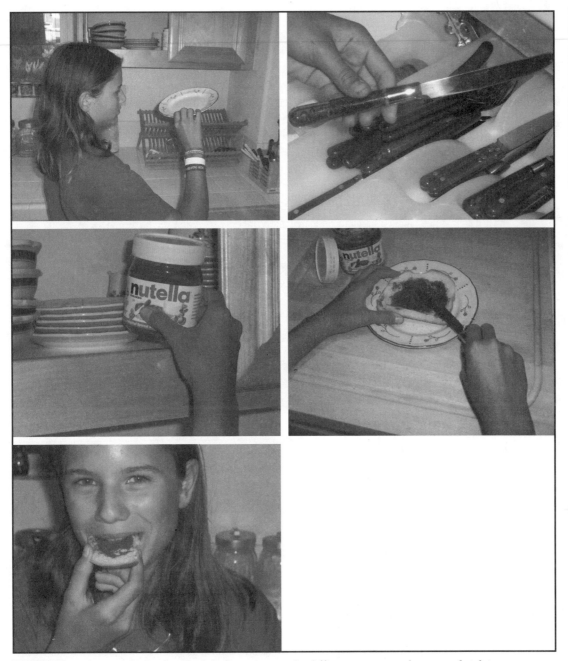

FIGURE 7.17. A photographed mini-schedule demonstrates the different steps in making a sandwich.

- Once the child has completed the sequence, he or she returns the used items to the sink, cabinet, or finish box.
- The child takes the next picture from his or her daily planner and begins the next activity.

Variation

This task can be made more or less difficult by reducing the number of pictured steps or by making it a backward chain:

The child cuts a ready-made sandwich and then eats it.
The child puts peanut butter on the bread, cuts the bread, and then eats it.
The child gets the peanut butter himself or herself, puts it on the bread, cuts the bread, and then eats it.

Task Example 2: Understanding Adjectives

- The child is prompted to select the picture of a reinforcer from his or her communication book and attach it to a long, empty Velcro strip.
- Ten pictures or word cards showing everyday items and their attributes on separate pictures (e.g., *brown* shoes, *wet* washcloth, *five* pencils) are attached to the Velcro strip, creating a sequence of adjective–noun phrases.
- This sequence starts with the written instruction "Get the ..."
- After getting the correct item, the child is prompted to put it and the corresponding pictures in the finish box.
- The child is then prompted to continue retrieving items from the picture sequence.
- If the child is incorrect, the therapist prompts silently.
- When the child has followed all pictured instructions, thereby emptying the picture strip, he or she is allowed to exchange the picture of the reinforcer for the real items or activity.

Variations

- The child should be able to recognize simple objects alone first, followed by simple adjectives, before both parts are put together in a task.
- In the beginning, it may be easier for the child if the actual items (e.g., brown shoes) are on the table directly in front of him or her. At a later stage, the child can retrieve the items from different locations.
- The number of components of the instructions can be increased, such as in a treasure hunt game: "Find the next cue under the *old photo* of yourself *upstairs in Ann's room.*"

Note

When the child is working on receptive language, natural reinforcers are highly motivating, as in a child retrieving items for a bike ride (see Figure 7.18).

Form 7.20 shows how these examples could be recorded using the blank data form for visual learning in Appendix 7.B.

Related Literature

Frost, L., & Bondy, A. (2002). *The picture exchange communication system.* Newark, DE: Pyramid Educational Products.

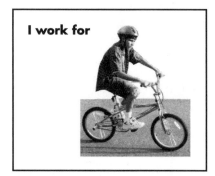

FIGURE 7.18. It is more motivating for children to link receptive commands to reinforcements, such as getting items (e.g., helmet, backpack) needed for riding a bike. (Source: *Picture This* [2003] www.silverliningmm.com)

Form 7.20. Example data form for visual learning method of teaching language comprehension skills.

		Instruction	
Target Skill	**Task**	**Verbal**	**Visual**
Unrelated multiple-step instructions	Name steps in making a sandwich	"Make a sandwich." (Name each step.)	Hand signs and pictured sequence of making a sandwich
Adjectives	Retrieve items	"Get the brown shoes."	Picture and hand sign

Child _____ Teacher _____

Skill Area Language Comprehension _____

Data Form for Visual Lear...

Hodgdon, L. A. (2000). *Visual strategies for improving communication.* Troy, MI: Quirk-Roberts.

McClannahan, L. E., & Krantz, P. J. (1999). *Activity schedules for children with autism: Teaching independent behavior.* Bethesda, MD: Woodbine House.

Mesibov, G., & Howley, M. (2003). *Assessing the curriculum for pupils with autistic spectrum disorders.* London: Fulton.

Active Communication and First Utterances

Section Overview

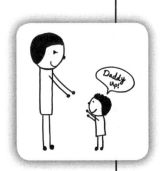

IMPORTANCE OF ACTIVE COMMUNICATION

Language is one of the most amazing skills children develop during their early years. With astonishing speed and seemingly little effort they expand their vocabulary, sentence structure, and use of language. They learn by interacting with their environment and experiencing and exploring objects long before using their names. An infant understands the concept of eating by mouthing edible and nonedible things. Concepts that are relevant and functional are mastered first, such as names of related people like *Mama, Papa,* or *Granny,* and names of important objects and activities like *milk, cookie, eat, water, bathe, play,* or *out.* Even the smartest babies do not say nonrelevant terms like *stock market* or *genes* as their first words (Bloom, 2000; Twachtman-Cullen, 2004).

Why train early active communication?

- Expression of requests and wishes
- Expression of affirmation, negation, refusal, and rejection
- Labeling of people, objects, and activities
- Greetings and farewells
- Expression of adjectives
- Description of past, present, and future
- Questions about objects, people, and locations
- Sharing events and experiences
- Social behavior and integration

Language development has a clear neurological basis, which obviously is disturbed in children with ASD. Their world tends to be less well organized as compared to that of their typically developing peers. For example, to understand that the word *cup* symbolizes a certain object and other like objects, a child has to associate seeing a cup with the spoken word. Because many young children with ASD are overselective, the association can easily go awry, such as when the child links the cup with the expression "Look here" or even with the spot on the table to which the mother pointed. The child also has to detach the idiosyncratic properties of his or her own cup (e.g., blue plastic cup with bear) and recognize the wide variety of cups available made of different colors, sizes, shapes, and material. At a later stage, she or he may need to understand that a cup is different from a glass and a mug, even though the cup serves a similar function. Because children with ASD have problems with associating crucial features to specific labels, they need training in matching and sorting, as previously discussed, plus specific language training.

To help children with autism learn to use language, therapists focus on training *pragmatics* in addition to standard programs on articulation, voice quality, vocabulary, and syntax. Pragmatics means "communication in context," referring to the various functions language serves in specific contexts (Camarata, 1996). See Figure 7.19.

> The word *dog* can mean "I want the dog" (requesting), "Don't take me near the dog!" (protesting), "Look, there is a dog" (alerting), or "Where is the dog?" (questioning).

The first utterances of typically developing children consist of requests, affirmations, refusals, rejections, greetings, farewells, descriptions, labels, and comments, followed by reports and questions. While these children develop a broad spectrum of communicative functions with ease, their autistic counterparts usually struggle with communication. Some of the nonverbal children resort to behaving disruptively to get their messages across: They want to be left alone, need a break, or require help with a difficult task. Sometimes they even communicate

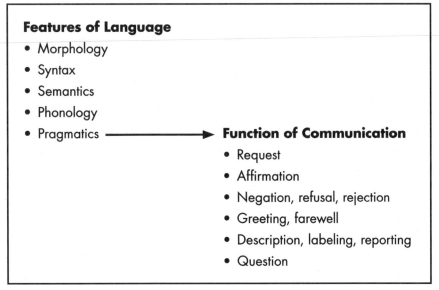

FIGURE 7.19. Pragmatics, or the function of communication, is a particular training focus for children with ASD.

unhappiness with severe tantrums, aggression, or self-injurious behavior. In such cases, the therapists should make teaching positive communicative alternatives a priority over a rigid pursuit of normal developmental sequences.

It has been shown that the development of alternative communication does reduce behavior problems. In one study, a behavior analysis demonstrated that some children echo utterances that they do not understand. Once these children learned to say, "I don't know" whenever an unknown object was presented, their echolalia was reduced (Schreibman & Carr, 1978). For children who tend to get upset and have a "meltdown" in demanding situations, learning to express "Help" or "I need a break" are logical alternatives.

Many children in the autism spectrum with higher IQs have age-appropriate or even advanced language skills but fail to say the right thing to the right person in the right setting in the right way. Some have odd posture and abnormal eye contact and may continuously get too close to the interaction partner. Others may not take turns but engage in lengthy monologues, ignoring the obvious boredom or frustration of the listener. To make these children competent communicators, therapists and others must teach the subtleties of communicative exchanges. This obviously is no easy undertaking because communication, cognition, and social skills are closely intertwined.

QUESTIONS FOR EVALUATING A CHILD'S SKILLS

Informal observations give a first impression of a child's abilities and problems with verbal and nonverbal communication. The following questions should be asked:

Questions that help determine the best way for a child to learn

- Does the child communicate by handing you objects, pushing your hand to desired items, or pointing?

(continues)

- Is the child able to imitate sounds, words, or sentences?
- Does the child name people, objects, or activities?*
- Does the child make requests?*
- Does the child affirm, protest, or reject?*
- Does the child use hand signs or gestures such as "bye-bye"?
- Does the child communicate through pictures or word-cards or by writing/typing?
- Does the child describe, comment, or alert you to things?*
- Does the child imitate communication in response to questions or spontaneously?
- Does the child use adjectives or adverbs?*
- How long are your child's utterances (e.g., one word, two words, three words)?*
- Does the child use social scripts appropriately (e.g., "help," "thanks," "please")?*

*Note. Specify if the child communicates verbally or nonverbally.

Developmental Levels for Early Active Communication

First communicative utterances tend to be aimed at either requesting something or protesting against something or somebody (Schuler, 1989). Many children with ASD do not develop beyond making these basic expressions. They are not able to communicate for social purposes such as alerting, informing, commenting, or asking questions (Wetherby & Prutting, 1989). For some children, unintelligible speech can hinder successful communication. Training of articulation may be required (Camarata, 1996). Verbal children with ASD often do not show much interest in communication and they lack spontaneous speech. They may answer questions but do not initiate or hold a true conversation. Some repeat utterances in an echolalic manner; others do so only when they do not understand what has been said. Even high-functioning children with ASD often fail to understand idioms, abstract language, and hidden meaning and need specific instruction on how to do so.

Because of the qualitative impairments of children with ASD in communication, the development of language and nonverbal utterances is a strategic masterpiece. Besides the normal developmental sequence, therapists must consider the child's individual interests and her or his optimal communication mode.

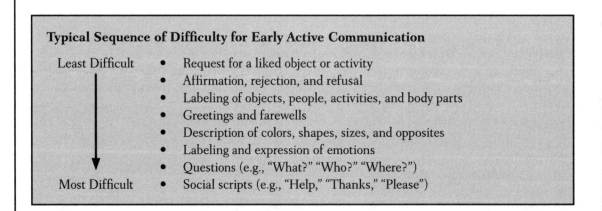

Typical Sequence of Difficulty for Early Active Communication

Least Difficult
- Request for a liked object or activity
- Affirmation, rejection, and refusal
- Labeling of objects, people, activities, and body parts
- Greetings and farewells
- Description of colors, shapes, sizes, and opposites
- Labeling and expression of emotions
- Questions (e.g., "What?" "Who?" "Where?")

Most Difficult
- Social scripts (e.g., "Help," "Thanks," "Please")

Prior to their first birthday, typically developing infants have learned various ways to communicate their needs. They alert others to their hunger, thirst, wet diapers, or loneliness by fussing or crying, while cooing and smiling indicate that they are well fed and happy. Even 6-month-old infants exhibit agitation in situations aimed at provoking jealousy (Hart, Jones, & Field, 2003). From 6 to 10 months, they start babbling, producing a variety of vowel and consonant sounds and even some combinations. They actively participate in simple interactive games, such as peekaboo, showing turn-taking behavior and communicative initiative. They indicate by stretching their arms up that they would like to be picked up and protest by facial expression and whining that their mother should not leave (Johnson-Martin et al., 1990). They point to objects and events initially to indicate their needs (i.e., proto-imperative pointing) and some time later to alert others (i.e., proto-declarative pointing; Mundy et al., 1994).

Between 12 and 18 months, most typical children use their first words and conventional gestures such as "bye-bye." A short time later, around their second birthday, they usually have about 25 to 50 active words, including object and action labels as well as names of people. Two-word sentences tend to occur around 24 months and three-word utterances at about 36 months. At this age, the first question, "What's that?" often seems to control all conversations and can frustrate even the calmest parents. A year later, the child is able to ask a variety of questions, form embedded sentences, and talk about experiences and past events (Kiphard, 1996).

Parents of infants later diagnosed with autism often note that their children have a restricted sound repertoire, do not babble, and do not develop first words or gestures at the expected age. Neither do their infants follow their gaze nor their pointing gesture. Some children use pointing, but tend to do so only to indicate their wishes and not to alert their parents to new events or exciting observations.

Parents of children with Asperger syndrome, on the other hand, often are surprised to witness the development of advanced vocabulary and complex sentence structures in their children. Still, these youngsters are far from being competent communicators. Some engage in monologues about their unique interests, ignoring any questions, objections, or signs of disinterest by the listener. Their stilted monologues have given them the dubious description of "little professors." They do not consider the prior knowledge, beliefs, or interests of the listener and do not seem interested in the listener's opinion.

The following STEP training aims to help children on both ends of the autism spectrum. Based on the described impairments, the teaching targets are organized according to pragmatics. The next section presents more complex utterances and expanded vocabulary. At all levels, the support of experienced speech–language pathologists, psychologists, behavior therapists, and teachers and close cooperation with parents are highly recommended.

How To Conduct the Training

Communication training can be conducted in one-to-one and small-group situations, at the computer, during a table task, or in everyday activities. If children are nonverbal and lack the prerequisites for active communication, intensive behavioral intervention is usually necessary. Vocabulary, articulation, and specific language structures can be trained in table and computer settings. At a more advanced level of communication development, role-play, play-groups, and more normalized training opportunities in inclusive settings can be provided (Camarata, 2001). As with all choices regarding therapy methods, the characteristics of the individual child and the specific therapy goal should be taken into consideration.

Training that follows the discrete trial format is usually conducted at a table with the therapist or parent sitting opposite the child. In the beginning, desirable objects are presented with the instruction "Say 'am/mamam' [for "eat"]/eat." If the child responds correctly, she or he is praised and receives the food item. In the course of training, the therapist requests increasingly more difficult imitations from the child. For example, for *ball*, the therapist accepts "b...," then "ba...," and finally, "ball." If the child wants to be lifted up in the air, the therapist accepts "u…," then "up." Once the child has mastered an imitation, the therapist presents the object or gesture without giving a model. Now the child is expected to respond to the question, "What do you want?" Because the response is no longer imitated, but elicited, it is called a *respondent request*. In the next step, the question is faded and the child must request without aid, exhibiting spontaneous speech (see Figure 7.20). This teaches the child to request objects or activities independently. When the child needs help, the therapist prompts at the previous level. Learning steps are mastered when a child performs a behavior either on two consecutive sessions at 80% or above or once at 90% or above. The behavior then has to be generalized to other people, materials, and settings.

In precision teaching, language programs stress the automatic production of sounds, syllables, words, and sentences. Many children with ASD have acquired some rudimentary language skills but apply them only on rare occasions. Speaking seems to require an enormous effort on the part of these children because language is not automatically available. This is similar to a person's reluctance to speak a foreign language today that was learned in school some time ago and never used daily (Bernard-Opitz, 2005). Through intensive practice of increasingly faster imitation and labeling exercises, the amount of effort required for language is reduced and spontaneity is increased.

Natural teaching and experience-based learning paradigms stress motivation and spontaneity in a child's teaching. Some children obviously need incentives to learn new vocabulary. Fortunately, their motivation increases when mastered words are interspersed with new and difficult ones (R. Koegel et al., 1988). In addition to receiving the object that was correctly named, children are motivated by being praised and seeing improvement over small time periods. Generalization training can be incorporated from the beginning of training using the strategy of multiple examples, in which several objects illustrate one concept. For example, the word *ball* is trained with various balls instead of just one, including a softball, a ping-pong ball, a basketball, a tennis ball, and a small rubber ball. The child learns to associate balls of different colors, materials, and sizes with one concept.

Spontaneous communication has been facilitated through the interrupting behavior chains strategy (Goetz et al., 1985). Actions with continual motion, such as walking up and down stairs, swinging, eating, drinking, assembling or disassembling a puzzle, threading beads, or taking objects out of a bag, are interrupted to give the child an incentive to request the continuation of the chain.

> During lunch, the parent or therapist labels the action as the child moves the spoon to his or her mouth, such as, "eat … eat … eat." Suddenly, the adult interrupts the movement of the spoon. When the child imitates "eat," she or he is allowed to continue eating.

An experience-based learning strategy that can motivate communication is called *mild distress in teaching*. Here, children are confronted with settings that motivate them to either solve a problem or request a change.

Step 1: Imitative utterances ("Ball")

Step 2: Respondent utterances ("What is this?")

Step 3: Spontaneous utterances (No verbal prompt)

FIGURE 7.20. Language training moves from imitative to respondent to spontaneous utterances.

On the way from class to the bus, a child expects to make the usual right turn. Instead, she or he is guided left by the teacher. Only when the child indicates that something is wrong is she or he allowed to walk the usual way. While nonverbal communication, such as pulling the teacher, is accepted in the beginning of this exercise, later steps require increasingly more differentiated communication, such as the child shaking his or her head or saying, "no" or "wrong way."

Many common situations can be used to entice children into spontaneous communication, such as getting less-preferred or even disliked food or drink, puzzle pieces that do not fit, unexpected items such as pencils in the lunchbox or a ladle for desert, or cold water in the bath instead of the anticipated warm water. If a child does not communicate appropriately in these situations, the therapist or parent gives immediate prompts so the child does not get unduly frustrated but learns the appropriate way to communicate.

Some children are better able to communicate through visual systems, such as pictures, word cards, or hand signs. It has been shown that children can learn to initiate communication and even develop speech through the *Picture Exchange Communication System* (PECS; Charlop-Christy et al., 2002). PECS is based on a simple idea: In exchange for passing the picture of a liked item to the interaction partner, the child receives the pictured item.

In PECS training, the parent or therapist and the child sit opposite each other with an assistant behind the child. A liked item, such as a cookie, is placed just out the child's reach while a picture of the cookie is within reach. When the child tries to grab the cookie, the assistant redirects the child's hand to the photo and prompts her or him to place it in the open hand of the therapist. The therapist praises the child, commenting on the request (e.g., "You want the cookie"). The procedure is repeated several times, fading the prompt of the stretched-out hand. Later, the child has to request the therapist's attention and alert him to the picture. Over the course of training, other language functions, such as descriptive utterances and longer sentences, are developed (Frost & Bondy, 2002).

Children who are good at imitating and who have developed spontaneous gestures are often good candidates to learn communication through hand signs (Bernard-Opitz et al., 1992; Carr, 1982). Comparable to teaching verbal requests, training of hand signs starts with imitations. Once this is mastered, children learn to show a sign in response to liked items and eventually can make spontaneous requests. Over the course of training, various language functions and increased sentence length are developed.

No matter the chosen strategy, the learned behavior must be generalized to the everyday environment of the child. The following training sequence offers a guideline for the development of a child's first verbal and nonverbal utterances. Utterances were selected based on the following criteria:

- Activities favored by many children with autism, such as toys with sensory appeal (e.g., battery-operated toys)
- Liked objects and activities (e.g., eating, jumping)
- Special interests (e.g., computer)
- Common activities (e.g., brushing teeth, blowing nose)
- Developmental sequence of language gains in typical children
- Ease with which the expressions are articulated

Therapists should consider children's social contexts (e.g., family preference, culture) for items such as food, toys, clothes, and activities. While the first utterances listed in the exercises that follow are aimed mainly at children with language skills below the age of 3 years, more advanced training goals are summarized in the next section of the chapter.

TRAINING PROGRAM OVERVIEW

Form 7.21 outlines training programs to develop active communication skills. The listed teaching targets should be assessed prior to the intervention and following a period of training. Once the child's profile of skills, learning channels, and interests has been determined, the therapist can select one of the four subsequent teaching methods. A reproducible copy of the form can be found in Appendix 7.A.

Before beginning exercises with a child, the therapist should note that expressive language is based on language comprehension. Therefore, this section on active communication must be considered in conjunction with the previous section on comprehension. The following section on expanded communication continues this training. As always, the sequence of tasks should be used as a guideline and should be adapted to the individual child.

EXAMPLES FOR DISCRETE TRIAL FORMAT

Example Task 1: Request for Object or Activity

- The child and therapist sit facing each other.
- The therapist holds up a requested object or a part thereof (e.g., a puzzle piece) and asks, "What do you want?"
- If the child responds correctly (e.g., says the word or an approximation, gives the picture, makes the hand sign), she or he is praised and receives the item.
- If she or he does not respond or makes an incorrect response, she or he is prompted (e.g., the therapist models the word, shows the mouth position, models the hand sign, or points to the correct picture).

Form 7.21. Overview of the STEP training programs for active communication; can be used as a pretest and posttest.

STEP Training Overview:
Active Communication

Child _____ Teacher _____

❑ Pretest ❑ Posttest

Communication Function	Task	Date Tested	Child's Response		Notes
			+	−	
Request	Therapist: "What do you want?" "Who do you want? "Which one do you want? Child: "I want _____."				
Objects					
Food and drink	Chips, cookie, M&M, banana, rice, juice, milk				
Toys	Bubbles, ball, balloon, yo-yo, sand, water, television, computer				

Variation

The child is allowed to choose among objects and pictures (e.g., "Which one do you want?").

Note

The child is prompted throughout the day to communicate her or his requests. The spontaneity of utterances is considered more important than the specific form of the communication.

Example Task 2: Affirming, Rejecting, and Denying

- The therapist shows the child a liked or disliked object such as candy or a piece of cauliflower.
- The therapist asks, "Do you want this?"
- If the child nods her or his head or says, "yes," she or he receives the object.
- If the child shakes her or his head or says, "no," the object is put aside.
- If there is an obvious discrepancy between the child's communication and her or his nonverbal behavior, such as shaking her or his head but grabbing for the object, the trial is considered incorrect, and the child does not receive the item.
- In this case, and whenever the child fails to respond, the therapist uses a prompt (e.g., modeling the respective communication, providing physical guidance).

Variation

At later stages of therapy, "yes" or "no" responses can be elicited for the following:

- Object name (e.g., "Is it a ball?")
- Action (e.g., "Does the boy ride a bike?")
- Person (e.g., "Is this your brother?")

Notes

- In general, "yes" and "no" utterances to request or reject objects are easier to make than utterances for descriptive statements.
- Rejected objects are used only once and are put aside upon the child's rejection.
- A possible task setup for this exercise is presented in Figure 7.21.

Form 7.22 shows how these examples could be recorded using the blank data form for discrete trial format in Appendix 7.B.

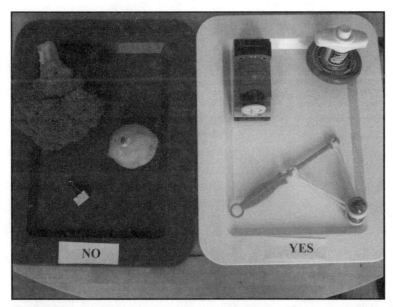

FIGURE 7.21. In the beginning of a "yes–no" training, clear task set-up is helpful to answer the question "Do you want this?" correctly.

Form 7.22. Example data form for discrete trial format method of teaching active communication.

Data Form for Discrete Trial

Child _____ Teacher _____

Skill Area <u>**Active Communication**</u> _____

In addition to recording the child's performance, indicate specifics about the task setup, s
schedule. Try to conduct about 10 trials per date and five sessions per week. Note that if the
Plot data on daily learning graphs.

Target Skill	Task Setup		Prompt	Consequence
	Material or Task	**Instruction**		
Request for objects	Liked object	"What do you want?"	Model word; show picture; make hand sign	Pass requested item; allow access to requested person; engage in requested activity
Expression of ~~~mation~~	Liked or disliked ob~~~	"Do you want th~~~	Nod or shake ~~~ay, "ye~~~	Pass or withdraw ~tem

Related Literature

Leaf, R., & McEachin, J. (1999). *A work in progress.* New York: DRL Books.

Maurice, C., Green, G., & Luce, S. C. (1996). *Behavioral intervention for young children with autism.* Austin, TX: PRO-ED.

EXAMPLES FOR PRECISION TEACHING

Example Task 1: Labeling Objects, People, and Activities

- The therapist arranges 6 to 10 objects or pictures in a circle.
- The therapist sets the timer for 20 seconds.
- The therapist asks the child, "What is this?," pointing to pictures in random sequence.
- The therapist acknowledges correct responses.
- If the child makes a mistake, the therapist quietly corrects.
- When the timer rings, the therapist records the numbers of correct and incorrect responses.
- If the child has improved her or his previous performance, she or he receives a token.
- After collecting three tokens, she or he receives a reinforcer.

Variation

- Several representatives of one word, such as different spoons or cups, can be displayed.
- Objects that the child can label fluently can be mixed with those that he or she is learning.
- The therapist starts out pointing to the objects or pictures in a fixed (e.g., clockwise) sequence and later switches to pointing randomly.

Note

See–say tasks have a fluency rate of about 50 to 55 responses per 1 minute, but the therapist should consider the individual child.

Cross-Reference

The described exercises for see-say tasks should be conducted once the child has mastered hear-say and hear-do tasks.

Task Example 2: Greetings and Farewells

- Several children or adults sit or stand in a circle around the child.
- The child is asked to greet each person (e.g., "Look at the person and say 'hello' or 'hi'").
- The number of persons greeted within 30 seconds is counted.
- Positive responses, such as eye contact and greeting, are acknowledged by nodding and saying "uh-huh."
- When the child improves her or his performance compared to previous trials, she or he gets a token.
- Once the child has received three tokens, he or she may exchange them for a reinforcer.

Prerequisite

- The child should have mastered looking at people and greeting, but still needs to learn to greet spontaneously.

Variation

- The number of required greetings within a specified time unit can be increased successively until the child has reached the fluency goal, which can be determined by measuring the fluency of a comparable peer.
- At a later stage, the child learns to greet only people who look familiar, rather than strangers.
- The child learns to use various brief, culturally common greeting scripts (e.g., "How are you?" "How is it going?" "What's up?").

Form 7.23 shows how these examples could be recorded using the blank data form for precision teaching in Appendix 7.B.

Form 7.23. Example data form for precision teaching of active communication.

Child _____ Teacher _____

Skill Area **Active Communication** _____

| Target Skill | Task Setup | | Time Unit | Consequence | Le HI |
	Material or Task	Instruction			
Description and labeling		"What is this?"	Frequency in 20 seconds	Verbal confirmation of "Uh-huh" and head nods for correct replies; token for improved performance compared to previous trial	He
Greetings and farewells		"Say, 'hello,'" "Say, 'hi,'" "Say, 'bye-bye'"	Frequency in 30 seconds	Verbal confirmation of "Uh-huh" and head nods for correct replies; token	Hea

EXAMPLES FOR NATURAL AND EXPERIENCE-BASED TEACHING

Example Task 1: Requesting Objects or Actions

- The therapist comments on an activity the child is doing, such as walking upstairs, swinging, or eating a cookie, saying "Up, up, up," "Swing, swing," or "Eat, eat," respectively.
- After about three utterances of the word, the therapist interrupts the child's movement and looks at her or him expectantly.
- If the child communicates spontaneously (e.g., by eye contact, vocalization, gesture, picture, or word), she or he is allowed to continue the activity another two or three times.
- The therapist then interrupts again and waits for the child to communicate.

Variation

- The child is interrupted frequently during everyday activities, such as while bike riding, playing at the playground, and getting a bath (see Figure 7.22).
- Once the child attempts to communicate, she or he is allowed to continue her or his activity.
- Over the course of the training, increasingly more difficult communication is requested (e.g., from eye contact to gestures, pictures or vocalizations to words).

Example Task 2: Social Scripts—Requesting Help

- The therapist offers an interesting toy or liked food item in a tightly closed see-through container.
- The therapist asks the child, "Do you want this?"

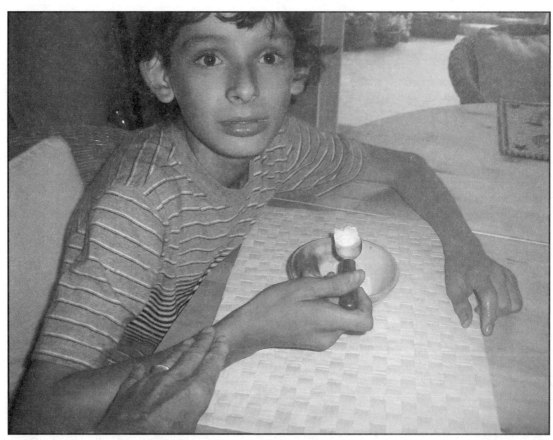

FIGURE 7.22. The child was interrupted while he was eating his ice cream and could continue only when he looked at his mother, who then commented, "Mmm, ice cream tastes good."

- If the child indicates an interest (e.g., says "yes" or grabs), she or he is handed the container.
- Because the child cannot open it, the therapist takes the container and waits for the child to request help.
- If the child does so, the therapist opens it immediately and passes it to the child.
- If the child does not respond, the therapist prompts the child to say, "Help," to pass the *help* card, or to make the *help* hand sign.

Variation

Objects of interest can be put into different bags or containers that have a variety of challenging fasteners (e.g., tape, zipper, thread, buttons). The containers are opened only when the child requests help from the therapist.

Table 7.5 provides examples of how natural teaching can be used to develop active communication skills. Form 7.24 shows a data form that can be used to record a child's responses to natural teaching. This form can be reproduced from Appendix 7.B.

Table 7.5
Examples of Ways Natural and Experience-Based Teaching Can Be Used To Develop Active Communication

Communicative Function	Task
Request for	
	Objects
Food and drink	Th: "What do you want?" Ch: "I want cookie."
Toys	Th: "What do you want?" Ch: "I want ball."
Clothing	Th: "What do you want?" Ch: "Take off shoes."
	Person/names
	Th: "Who wants an ice cream?" Ch: "I do," "Mommy does."
	Th: "Who do you want to play with?" Ch: "Grandpa," "Tommy."
	Actions
	Liked activities, such as eating, throwing toys into the bathtub, swinging, and jumping, are interrupted until the child labels each of them or requests the action.
	Th: "Swing, swing" (stops the child up in the air) "Again?" Ch: "Swing again!"
	Th: "What do you want?" Ch: "Play (or swing, slide, swim, ride, push, splash, throw)."
	Object features
	Th: "Do you want the big or small cookie (or the red or green apple, or the long or short train)?"
	Th: "Do you want one nut (or many nuts)?"

Table 7.5. *(Continued)*

Communicative Function	Task
Expression of Affirmation/ Rejection/Denial	**Objects** Th: "Do you want the apple (or ice cream or broccoli)?" Th: "Is this a towel (or soap, or CD, or pillow)?" **People** Th: "Shall Mom come?" "Do you want to play with Maria?" "Does Carlos watch TV?" "Does Papa wash the car?" **Actions** Th: "Do you want to roll the ball?" Th: "Is he combing his hair?" **Object features** Th: "Do you want a big or small cookie (or brown or yellow M&M)?" Th: "Is the beach towel wet or dry?"
Description/Labeling of Objects/Actions	"What is it?" "What do you see (or hear or keep or take or play with)?" / "This is a … / These are … / I see/eat (a) / play with …" / "What is in the bag/on the shelf/in the refrigerator?"
• Food/drink	Th: "What is happening?" Ch: "Eating cake."
• Toys	Th: "What are you playing with?" Ch: "Balloon (or book, puzzle, yo-yo, swing)."
• Household	Th: "What are you doing?" Ch: "Sitting (or washing or sleeping)."
• Utensils	Th: "What are you doing?" Ch: "Wiping (or cleaning, drying, coloring, painting)."
• Clothing	Th: "What is happening?" Ch: "Putting on shoes."
• Vehicles	Th: What are you doing?" Ch: "Riding bicycle."
• Locations	Th: "Where is Mama (or Papa or Kayla)?" "Mama is in the _____." Ch: "Garden (or pool or bath)." Th: "Where is the chocolate?" "The chocolate is behind the _____." Ch: "Box (or bag or pillow or bed)."
Persons • Names	Th: "Who is it?" "Who has the marble?" "Who wears a hat?" "Who reads a book?" "Who rides the skateboard?"
• Body parts	Th: "We put the lotion on your _____." "We wash your _____."
• Emotions	The therapist stresses emotions in everyday situations, during play and book readings, while watching videos and looking at photos. Th: "You are so _____." Ch: "… hungry (or thirsty or tired or happy or sad)." Th: "Sunni is crying. She is very _____." Ch: "sad."

(continues)

Table 7.5. *(Continued)*

Communicative Function	Task
Actions/Functions of Objects/Body Parts	Th: (sings) "This is the way we clap our hands, clap our hands, clap our _____ (Continues with "stamp our feet" and "nod our head"). Ch: "hands (or feet or head)." Th: "What are we doing?" Ch: "Cooking (or coloring or running or jumping)."
Animals	Th: "What animal is it?" "What do you see?" "This is a _____." "Oh no, there comes a _____." "We color the _____." Ch: "Dog (or cat or cow or goat or lion)."
Greeting/goodbye	In regular and play settings, greetings and farewells are practiced with peers, dolls, animals, and puppets, at doors, curtains, and puppet theaters. Th: "Hello" "How are you?" "Bye-bye."
Description of Object Features	Th: "The balloon (or car or Lego brick) is _____." Th: "Which car (or balloon or cookie or sausage) do you want?" Ch: "Red (or blue or big or small)." Th: "Do you want a little or a lot of the soup?" Ch: "A little," "A lot."
Questions	Interesting objects (e.g., noisemakers, wind-up toys) are hidden and the child is prompted to ask for them. "Ask about the bag (or cookie or flashlight)!"
• "What?"	"What is it?" "What's inside?"
• "Who?"	"Who has it?"
• "Where?"	"Where is it?"
Social Scripts	
• "Please/thank you/ thanks"	Objects are withheld until the child says, "Please (or thank you or thanks)," or until the child requests help to get access to liked items.
• "Help (me)"	

EXAMPLES FOR VISUAL LEARNING

Example Task 1: Communication of a Request— Hand Sign for *More*

- The therapist shows the child a bowl of a liked food item (e.g., cereal, raisins, nuts, Smarties, M&Ms).
- The therapist gets the child's attention and offers her or him one of the food items.
- After the child takes one item, the therapist closes the container to prevent the child from helping herself or himself to the other food items.
- The therapist asks, "Do you want more?"
- If the child signs or says, "More" or "yes," or passes the appropriate picture or word card, she or he is allowed to take another item.

Form 7.24. Blank data form for natural and experience-based teaching of active communication.

	Task Setup		
Target Skill	**Material or Task**	**Instruction**	**Consequence**

Data Form for Natural and Experience...

Child _____   Teacher _____

Skill Area _Active Communication_ _____

- If the child fails to respond, she or he is prompted by the therapist's modeling the sign or pointing to the card.
- The procedure is repeated about 10 times.

Variation

Toys that have several pieces or that need to be assembled also can be used, such as marbles for a marble drop, blocks for a tower, pieces for a puzzle, or tracks for a train.

Notes

- The child should improve his or her responses over the session(s).
- Over the course of a session, hand signs and words should become more similar to the therapist's model.
- While modeled hand signs or words can be reinforced in the beginning, the therapist should expect direct answers to the questions in later trials, without the therapist modeling the sign "more."
- Assistance given during the exchange also should be faded during the session(s).
- The distance between the therapist and the child, and the child and the picture, should increase with the child's progress (Frost & Bondy, 2002).
- The selection of a communication system and the choice of utterances should be based on the prerequisites of the individual child.
- For some children, hand-sign communication is easier, while others communicate better through pictures and word cards.
- Some children pick up general utterances such as "more," "eat," "drink," and "play" faster, while others find it easier to acquire more specific words such as "banana" or "water."

Example Task 2: Labeling Everyday Objects With "I See ..."

Prior to starting the training, the child selects the picture of a reinforcer from her or his picture album.

Step 1

- The therapist places 10 known objects on the table (e.g., crayon, car).
- The corresponding pictures are placed in a PECS booklet in front of the child.
- On the front page of the book, a sentence strip indicates, "I see [blank Velcro space]."
- The child picks up a specific object such as a crayon and places its corresponding picture on the sentence strip.
- She or he passes the completed strip of "I see crayon" to the therapist.
- The therapist places the crayon in the finish box.
- The therapist praises the child enthusiastically (e.g., "Good! You see a crayon").
- The therapist takes the crayon picture off the sentence strip and passes the strip back to the child, encouraging the child to "tell me more."
- When all objects are labeled and the table is empty, the child receives a reinforcer, such as a previously determined activity. (Figure 7.23 shows an example of this task.)

Step 2

- Child and therapist walk alongside a wall that has various items attached to it with Velcro, such as an empty cookie box, a small sponge ball, or an empty bubbles container.
- The child is instructed to pass the therapist a sentence strip that says, "I see a ...," and then point to what she or he sees on the wall.
- If the child needs assistance, the therapist combines pointing to an item on the wall with a surprised sound: "Wow! You sure saw crayons!"
- When the child points appropriately, she or he is praised and receives a functional reinforcer such as a real cookie for pointing to the cookie box.

Step 3

The child is asked to describe objects in the room with her or his PECS, pointing to an object, looking for the corresponding picture, and passing the completed sentence strip to the therapist.

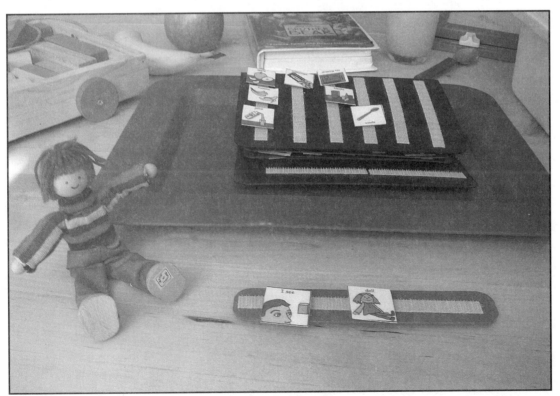

FIGURE 7.23. In this task, the child describes what he or she sees with the PECS sequence "I see the doll." (Source: www.pecs.com)

Form 7.25. Example data form for visual learning method of teaching active communication.

Data Form for Visual Lear

Child _____   Teacher _____

Skill Area ___Active Communication___

Target Skill	Task	Instruction	
		Verbal	**Visual**
Request for object	Ask for more food items	"Do you want more?"	Child shows hand sign, picture, or wor cards
Description and labeling	Name object	"What is this?" "What do you see (or hear or feel)?"	PECS card or sentence strip: "I see _____"

Variation

- The therapist trains the task with hand signs and word cards.
- The child takes objects from a surprise box or bag (e.g., box or bag with Styrofoam pieces and small, hidden objects) and labels them.
- A similar task setup can be done with "I feel" or "I hear."

Form 7.25 shows how these examples could be recorded using the blank data form for visual learning in Appendix 7.B.

Related Literature

Camarata, S. M. (1996). On the importance of integrating naturalistic language, social intervention, and speech-intelligibility training. In L. K. Koegel, R. L. Koegel, & G. Dunlap (Eds.), *Positive behavioral support*. Baltimore: Brookes.

Frost, L., & Bondy, A. (2002). *The picture exchange communication system*. Newark, DE: Pyramid Educational Products.

Hodgdon, L. A. (2000). *Visual strategies for improving communication*. Troy, MI: QuirkRoberts.

Mesibov, G., & Howley, M. (2003). *Assessing the curriculum for pupils with autistic spectrum disorders*. London: Fulton.

Schopler, E., Reichler, R. J., Bashford, A., Lansing, M. D., & Marcus, L. M. (1990). *The psychoeducational profile–revised*. Austin, TX: PRO-ED.

Expanded Communication

Section Overview

Importance of Expanded Communication

Questions for Evaluating a Child's Skills

Developmental Levels for Expanded Communication

How To Conduct the Training

Training Program Overview

Examples for Discrete Trial Format

Examples for Precision Teaching

Examples for Natural and Experience-Based Teaching

Examples for Visual Learning

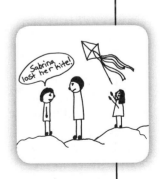

IMPORTANCE OF EXPANDED COMMUNICATION

Once children are able to use about 50 one-word utterances, vocabulary and sentence length can be expanded and grammatical structures introduced. Comparable to the development of first words, children must learn to use various language functions. Although requesting is an important function, it is only one of several that need to be developed; the training of spontaneous speech is equally important.

Why train expanded communication?

- Expansion of spontaneous communication
- Expansion of expressive vocabulary (e.g., food, household objects, school objects, professions, vehicles, utensils, relatives, calendar months)
- Expansion of descriptive words (e.g., adjectives, comparatives, associations, adverbs)
- Comprehension and expression of categories and subcategories
- Expansion of grammatical structures (e.g., singular, plural, past, present, future, pronouns, conjunctions, declensions)
- Expansion of language functions (e.g., greeting, request, instruction, command, comment, interjection, correction)
- Expansion of sentence length and complexity (e.g., two-, three-, and more-word sentences, embedded sentences)
- Training of sayings (e.g., "keep it up," "zip your mouth," "hang on," "hang in there," "be on your toes," "he's pulling your leg," "don't beat around the bush")
- Conversation (e.g., topics, instructions, questions)

To become competent communicators, children have to learn several thousand words. These include common expressions, such as those related to frequently used household, school, and play items, and less-common vocabulary, such as that related to advanced body parts, vehicles, traffic signs, types of relatives, and sayings. Over time, children also learn to comprehend and actively use adjectives, adverbs, prepositions, and comparatives. By doing so they can ask successfully for the "biggest cookie," or understand that "the book is on the lower shelf on the right-hand side." They learn to divide time into months, weeks, days, and hours to the point where they can understand that "Next Monday there is no P.E." Interjections such as "Okay" or "Alright," "Done Deal," "Agreed," "Super," "Cool," "Great," and "Wait" are common exchanges in school and homes and often are not understood by children with ASD. In general, these children have to be explicitly taught how to understand and apply these terms.

When a person with ASD meets someone new, the first few seconds often determine her or his acceptance. If nonverbal features, such as clothing, posture, facial expression, and gesture, and verbal communication match those of the peers, positive relations are more likely to begin. A child with ASD who has learned, in therapy, to greet people with a handshake or a "Good morning" is likely to be considered unusual or, even worse, a "nerd" by his or her typical peers.

As early as kindergarten, it is expected that children will know their age, address, family, teachers, and friends and will be able to answer questions accordingly. Children should know basic functions of objects (e.g., "What do you use for eating [or writing]?"), materials (e.g., "What is the shirt [or shoes or paper] made of?"), locations (e.g., "What belongs in the kitchen [or refrigerator or zoo]?"), professions (e.g., "What does a police officer [or hairdresser] do?"), animals (e.g., "Where does the egg [or milk] come from?"), and problem solving (e.g., "What do you need when it's raining [or when you have lost something]?").

When teaching communication, therapists should have access to picture or photo libraries and schedule programs such as Boardmaker (www.mayer-johnson.com), Do2learn (www.do2 learn.com), Picture This Pro (www.silverliningmm.com), or IconTalk (www.icontalk.com). In addition, parents and teachers may find commercial flash cards, picture books, photo libraries, and specialized software useful (e.g., see www.laureatelearning.com, www.palsprogram.com, www .teachtown.com). Self-made digital photos or video clips also can provide visual support for sequencing past or future events. A variety of assistive devices have helped children with ASD communicate more effectively (e.g., www.dynavoxsys.com). Pocket PCs are being developed to store digital libraries that are relevant to individual children and that assist with vocal output and communication (Leroy, Chuang, Huang, & Charlop-Christy, 2005).

This section gives an overview of programs for training expanded communication. The presented tasks represent only a small sample of this teaching area. Because a detailed curriculum for expanded communication goes beyond the scope of this book, the reader is advised to consult additional readings (Blank et al., 2000; Braun, 2002; Freeman & Dake, 1997; Hodgdon, 2000; Partington & Sundberg, 1998; Quill, 2002). In addition to following the described program, therapists should seek the help of experienced language specialists.

QUESTIONS FOR EVALUATING A CHILD'S SKILLS

To develop successful communication in children with ASD, therapists must choose motivating settings, interesting topics, and communication systems that match children's needs. Many children with good visual discrimination skills benefit either from the *Picture Exchange Communication System* (PECS) or hand-sign training. Compared to speech, both of these methods have fewer prerequisites and often lead to spontaneous communication within the first hours of therapy. If children are able to say a few words, but are having a hard time expanding their repertoires, alternative communication systems should be considered (Frost & Bondy, 2002).

Questions that help determine the best way for a child to learn

- Does the child communicate through words, pictures, word cards, or hand signs?
- Can strangers understand the child?
- Does the child use at least 50 communicative utterances?
- Does the child use various communicative functions, such as requests, descriptions, affirmations, negations, and questions?
- Does the child communicate spontaneously?
- Can the child follow and use multiple-word utterances?
- Does the child participate in conversations by making comments or brief interjections?
- Can the child make comments that relate to the topic at hand?
- Can the child talk about certain topics?
- With whom does the child communicate best and in what setting?
- Can the child form sequences with beads, patterns, numbers, and pictures?
- Can the child report past events in the correct sequence?
- Can the child plan future events?
- Does the child have a basic knowledge of food, professions, vehicles, and animals?
- Is the child able to hold a conversation?

To expand a child's communication, the therapist should consider what person, setting, and topic elicit the child's best performance. While young children with ASD are frequently

> Interests and favorite topics can help to expand communication as long as they do not distract or overwhelm the child.

motivated by favorite food items, toys, and activities, children with more advanced skills often are fascinated by their special interests. Books, videos, computer programs, and toys on their favorite topics can motivate these children. Communication can be improved by incorporating Disney characters, Teletubbies, Pokemon, Spider-man, puppets, or figurines into training. Therapists, teachers, and parents have to ensure, though, that the topic interest does not overwhelm the child and that it can be used constructively to reach the main goal of expanding communication.

What vocabulary, grammatical structures, and language functions does the child use spontaneously? These questions can be answered by analyzing spontaneous language samples of the child. A taped assessment of the child's utterances can complement the STEP training sequence.

DEVELOPMENTAL LEVELS FOR EXPANDED COMMUNICATION

The language of typical children develops with breathtaking speed, especially during the preschool years. A typical 2-year old already has a vocabulary of 200 to 300 words and is able to communicate in one- to three-word utterances (Harris & Liebert, 1987). During this period children learn most morphemes, which are the smallest units of meaning, such as plural endings (Brown, 1979). Morphemes develop in a predictable sequence: Those with the most important meaning are acquired before those with less relevance. For example, because it is important for most children to be able to ask for "many cookies" instead of just one, to indicate that this is "my cookie" and not yours, and to understand that the cookies are "in the box" or "on the shelf," plural endings, possessive pronouns, and prepositions develop early.

The ability to create sequences is an important prerequisite for understanding past and future events, for recalling stories, and for developing the concepts of time, days, weeks, and months (Freeman & Duke, 1997). Children should be able to make sequences from color and shape patterns, numbers, and amounts before working on the calendar, the clock, or time. Three- to four-year-old typically developing peers usually have developed these skills without much instruction. Similarly, they are able to talk about the past and the future and to ask questions about the world around them (Goldhaber, 1986). By asking questions, they learn new terms and expand their knowledge about their environment. At a later stage, they learn to make *yes* and *no* utterances to answer questions such as, "Is this your brother?" While the word *and* is learned relatively fast, subordinate clauses and utterances with *because* or *as well as* are seen only in elementary school–age children.

When starting elementary school, children tend to have a passive vocabulary of 10,000 to 15,000 words and an active vocabulary of about 3,000 to 5,000 words (Braun, 2002). In many areas, their language can be compared to that of an adult.

It is more difficult to outline a typical sequence of difficulty for expanded communication than it is for early communicative utterances. Children's prerequisite skills, their idiosyncratic communicative problems, and the demands of different social settings vary widely. In children with ASD, the development of communication is less regular and often severely disturbed. Some children never use one- or two-word utterances, but right away talk in full sentences. Others repeat heard sentences like parrots, but still do not understand even simple words. While the training of expanded communication should follow the normal developmental sequence, therapists must consider the relevance of each teaching target for the individual child. For example, programs that train "Yes" and "No" often are highly functional for children with ASD and also less difficult for them to learn than other concepts.

For many children with ASD, spontaneity gets in the way of becoming a more competent communicative partner. A training sequence that moves systematically from imitative to respondent to spontaneous utterances is often necessary. Other children stumble over a lack of fluency in turn taking, reciprocal utterances, and appropriate social scripts. Developing more automatic performance is necessary in these cases.

Intelligibility and voice quality also can get in the way of social acceptance. Children who are difficult to understand or who talk in an unusual loudness, pitch, or intonation pattern may require a focus on normalizing their voices more than on expanded vocabulary or grammatical structures. In addition to training speech intelligibility, increasing the familiarity and acceptance of speech and providing augmentative devices have been shown to dramatically decrease behavior problems (Carr, 1982).

Therapists also must consider that even for typical children, developments within categories, such as body parts, are not homogeneous. The concepts of body parts such as *mouth, nose,* and *eyes* are usually acquired around age 2 years, while *shoulder, hip,* and *waist* are often known only at age 6 years. Frequently used adjectives such as *big* and *tall* and *little* and *small* are acquired faster than less frequent terms such as *shallow* and *deep.*

Expanding social scripts and conversational exchanges constitute another necessary puzzle piece. Both teaching targets have to be integrated with described programs on joint attention as well as the programs in the following section on social skill and play development.

How To Conduct the Training

Many questions surround the training sequence for language comprehension and expressive communication. For instance, teachers and parents often ask, Should comprehension always precede the production of speech? Obviously, comprehension and production are related, and typical children first understand language before they say their first words. However, active communication is still possible without the auditory processing of speech, as in the case of Helen Keller, although it is much more difficult.

Children with ASD usually go through comprehension training before they learn to engage in active communication. Sometimes a child acquires both the understanding and the expression in the same session. For example, learning the name of a body part and labeling it can go hand in hand. A child may point to his or her nose when the parent instructs, "Show me your nose." In the subsequent trial, the child is asked to give the word for nose when the parent, pointing appropriately, asks, "What is this?" For some children, this is the best way to learn expressive language, but others find the switch in instructions—from "Show me your nose" to "What is this?"—confusing. The exercises in this manual clearly separate the interventions, but it is up to the therapist to choose between a simultaneous and a sequential method. As always, the choice should be based on the responses of the individual child.

One of the methods known to be effective in expanding vocabulary, sentence structure, and communicative functions is the discrete trial format. This method's clear task structure, simple instructions, and unambiguous feedback can help develop complex communication skills.

Providing appropriate models, such as pictures and toys (see Figure 7.24), can also enhance complex communication (Blank et al., 2000). To trigger spontaneous utterances, the therapist can delay his or her verbal model systematically over the course of a session. The following example demonstrates this time-delay procedure:

MOTHER:	What did we buy?
MOTHER:	(without delay) Ice cream and apples.
CHILD:	Ice cream and apples.
MOTHER:	What did we buy?
MOTHER:	(with a 2-second delay) Ice cream and apples.

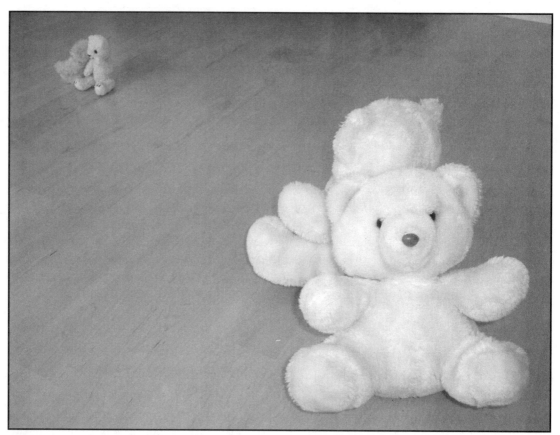

FIGURE 7.24. Stuffed toys can help develop complex language in children with ASD. Here, the therapist might say, "These teddy bears are big, while those are small."

During the course of the training, increasing time delays of 3, 4, and 5 seconds are inserted between the question and the model. In this way, the child learns to answer the questions directly without the adult's model:

> **MOTHER:**   What did we buy?
> **CHILD:**   Ice cream and apples.

At a later stage, the child is asked various questions in random order so that his or her answers become flexible and are no longer robotic (Bondy et al., 2002). As with other discrete trial format exercises, reinforcement is part of this training.

As indicated in this manual previously, precision teaching aims to make the production of communication fluent and automatic. The goal is for children to retain learned behaviors, use them spontaneously, and generalize them to everyday settings. According to the analyses of fluency rates of children between the ages of 18 months and 14 years, typical children can label 55 to 70 objects per minute (Fabrizio & Moors, 2003). Besides this general guideline, the therapist must consider individual learning rates when setting fluency aims.

> Preparing drinks and snacks, baking, and cooking are exceptional tasks to use for expanding speech and developing problem solving.

Training tasks in the area of natural and experience-based teaching are usually conducted during motivating situations, such as eating, playing, or engaging in hobbies or sports. Preparing drinks and snacks, baking, and cooking provide exceptional incentives to expand speech and develop problem solving (see Figure 7.25). "What do we need to make a chocolate drink?" ("Chocolate powder," "milk," "spoon, "cup"). "What do you want to do now?" ("Open the can," "take a spoon," "scoop chocolate powder").

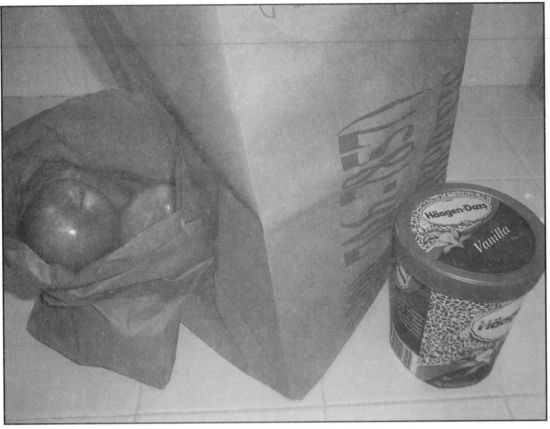

FIGURE 7.25. Talking about groceries helps to expand children's vocabulary, conversation skills, and even general knowledge.

In play settings, vocabulary and sentence structures can be taught and developed through the use of puppets, dolls, and animals. In storytelling, vocabulary, recall, and imagination can be enhanced, such as in the following example:

THERAPIST:	(pointing to a picture or doll of a witch) This is the mean ....
CHILD:	Witch.
THERAPIST:	(pointing to characters) She wants to ....
CHILD:	Catch Hansel and Gretel.
THERAPIST:	The children could hide behind the ....
CHILD:	Tree.

To develop fluid communication, therapists also can present models through earphones. The child hears and models appropriate replies, comments, or questions directly in the natural setting. This can be less confusing than imitating a live model directly and listening to the interaction partner simultaneously.

Robbie, 5 years old, had little communicative speech, but a strong tendency to echo heard utterances and a preference for technical gadgets. To develop Robbie's greetings, questions, and comments, his mother modeled appropriate speech into a microphone, which was relayed to Robbie through headphones. Using this method, the boy imitated the words necessary to greet his father whenever he came home from shopping. Robbie would follow his mother's model: "Hi, Dad, where have you been?" After learning that his dad had shopped at the supermarket, he repeated his mother's question: "What did you buy?" Next, he acknowledged the purchased goodies, again imitating his mother's model: "Wow, chocolate!" Through frequent repetition, Robbie learned to carry out this exchange spontaneously, without his mother's intervention.

Many programs designed to expand communication put the good visual skills of children with ASD to use. Pictures, symbols, or words cue the child to talk about the day, plan an exciting outing, comment on the play of a peer, or request a special sundae. Structures such as *first … and then …*, visual scripts for special topics such as movies, and syntax programs can be represented in pictures or writing (see Figure 7.26). In PECS, children use picture sequences to move from simple requests, such as, "want crayon," to more complex utterances, such as, "I want a red crayon, some paper, and scissors."

When children with ASD report on past events and future plans, pictures can serve as effective prompts (Hodgdon, 2000). The picture schedule shown in Figure 7.27 may help a child tell her parents about her day. In addition, souvenirs of past events, such as a bus ticket or leaves from the park, can help elicit recall and communication about past events.

From a trip to the zoo, 10-year-old Maggie brought home her entrance ticket, the zoo schedule, a postcard of the monkey exhibit, and a feather. With the help of these props, she successfully recounted the events of her special excursion.

Children with ASD are often overwhelmed when asked to recall events without tangible reminders. In *teaching tales* (Blank et al., 2000), two to four pictures are shown and teachers model sentences, questions, or comments (see Figure 7.28). To help with recall, a series of photographs of a special event can be put together for an individual child. Parents and therapists also may choose to draw their own story using simple stick figures.

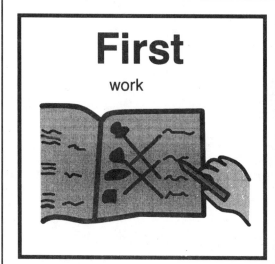 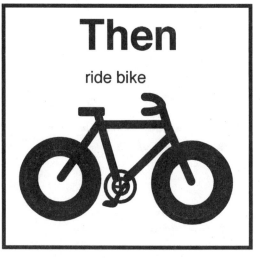

FIGURE 7.26. Example of "First … Then" construction. Visual cues, such as First and Then cards, can help children sequence and express their plans better.

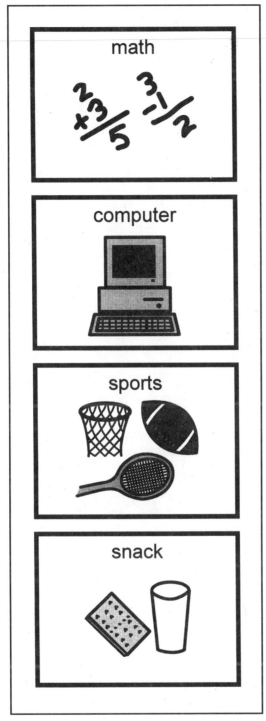

FIGURE 7.27. Pictures serve as effective prompts for children to learn expanded language, such as reporting on the day's activities.

Making recollections and plans requires that children be able to describe objects and events, know about matching objects to categories, and describe and sequence experiences. Again, visual prompts of pictures or words can help provide the structure children with ASD need for these skills (Freeman & Dake, 1997; see Figure 7.29). The following tables give examples.

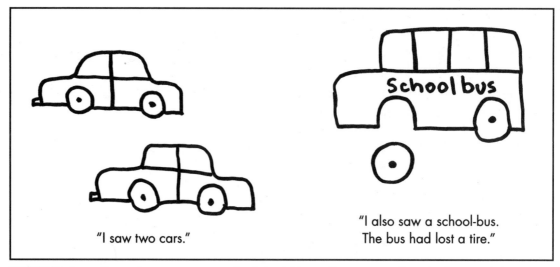

FIGURE 7.28. In teaching tales, pictures are used to help children tell stories. Recall can be facilitated through pictures of exciting events.

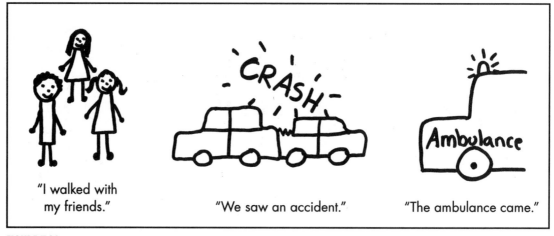

FIGURE 7.29. A visual prompt may help a child recall a car accident. Simple line-drawings can facilitate the early description of narratives.

Put the following words into the correct categories:

cabinet	horse	ball
yo-yo	train	noodles
cat	apple	rabbit
bread	chair	table

Animals	Food	Furniture	Toys

Name three things you need when you _____ .

Eat			
Dress yourself			
Play			

What do you think when you hear the word _____ ?

Birthday			
School			
Friends			

When a child begins the above exercises, the therapist can show books and drawings, play games, or provide written prompts, such as choices of possible answers. Next, the therapist can ask for the number of expected utterances. The instruction "Tell me three things that happened in school" is more likely to be answered than the question "How was school today?" In addition, some children are motivated by time limits, such as in the next table.

Within 1 minute, recall four things you did during the vacation (child dictates, writes, or selects pictures from array).

1.	3.
2.	4.

To enhance advanced communication in children with ASD, therapists must expand children's vocabulary, communicative functions, and conversation skills. The following STEP sequence shows therapy targets that have been useful with children and adults with ASD. This section builds on the previous one on early utterances and has close links to the upcoming section on play and social skills. Parents and therapists are again reminded that the described STEP training should be tailored to individual needs.

TRAINING PROGRAM OVERVIEW

Form 7.26 outlines training programs to develop expanded communication skills. The listed teaching targets should be assessed prior to the intervention and following a period of training. Once the child's profile of skills, learning channels, and interests has been determined, the therapist can select one of the four subsequent teaching methods. A reproducible copy of the form can be found in Appendix 7.A.

EXAMPLES FOR DISCRETE TRIAL FORMAT

Example Task 1: Communicative Function—Greeting, Farewell

- The child walks around the playground with the therapist.
- Whenever they meet a known person, the therapist greets, "Hello."

Form 7.26. Overview of the STEP training programs for expanded communication; can be used as a pretest and posttest.

STEP Training Overview:
Expanded Communication

Child _____ Teacher _____

❏ Pretest ❏ Posttest

Expanded Communication and Vocabulary Skills	Task Examples	Date Tested	Child's Response		Notes
			+	−	
Spontaneity					
Objects					
Food					
Toys					
Household items					
School					
Traffic					
Utensils					

- If the child does not follow the therapist's model, she or he is prompted (see next step).
- The therapist shows the child the word card "Hello."
- If the child responds correctly without the prompt, she or he is praised and receives a token.
- Prompted responses are only verbally reinforced.

Variations
- People on the playground can wear *Hello* buttons, giving the child visual prompts.
- Other scripts, such as "How are you?," can be practiced in a similar manner.

Example Task 2: Report Past and Future Events

Past Events
- The therapist and child do something interesting together (e.g., play with a wind-up toy, conduct a small experiment).
- The therapist sends the child to another interaction partner, instructing, "Tell him what you just did" (see Figure 7.30).
- If the child reports appropriately, she or he is praised.
- If the child needs help, the therapist prompts through a picture or a short written summary, which cues the child to report about the event to the new interaction partner.

Future Events
- The therapist plans something interesting with the child (e.g., search for batteries for a toy, feed an animal, conduct a small experiment).
- The therapist asks, "What do you want to do right now?"
- When the child states his intention, she or he is praised and allowed to engage in the planned activity.
- If the child needs help, the therapist prompts through a picture or short written summary.

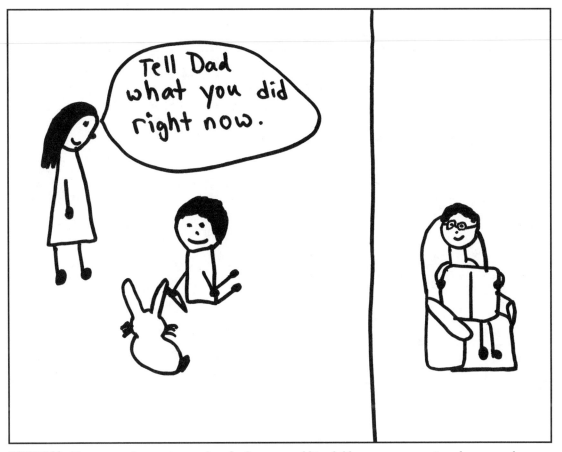

FIGURE 7.30. If events are interesting, such as feeding a pet rabbit, children are more motivated to report them.

Note

Souvenirs from recent events (e.g., pinecones from a walk in the forest, plastic plates from a snack at a fast-food restaurant, balloons from a birthday party) can elicit some details about these events.

Example Task 3: Social Scripts—"I Don't Know"

- A box with familiar and unfamiliar items is placed on the table.
- The therapist takes out one object after another, asking, "What is this?"
- When the child labels the object, she or he is praised and allowed to briefly handle the named object.
- When the child does not know the object, the therapist prompts, "I don't know."
- The child is praised for the imitation.
- Once the child anticipates the prompt, a prompt delay is introduced. That is, the therapist waits increasingly longer (e.g., 1, 2, 3 seconds) before providing the prompt.
- The child receives a token for appropriate "I don't know" utterances.
- Once the child has reached a specified number of tokens, she or he receives a reinforcer.

Variation

Instead of the verbal prompt, a word card can be used.

Form 7.27 shows how these examples could be recorded using the blank data form for discrete trial format in Appendix 7.B.

Form 7.27. Example data form for discrete trial format method of teaching expanded communication.

Data Form for Discrete Trial

Child _____   Teacher _____

Skill Area Expanded Communication _____

In addition to recording the child's performance, indicate specifics about the task setup, s⟍ schedule. Try to conduct about 10 trials per date and five sessions per week. Note that if the⟍ Plot data on daily learning graphs.

Target Skill	Task Setup		Prompt	Consequence
	Material or Task	Instruction		
Language functions: greetings and farewells	Saying "hello"	"Hello," "How are you?"	"Hello" with word card prompt	Praise; tokens
Past, present, future	"I'm taking a bath," "I fed the fish⟍	"Tell me what you just did," "⟍ you	Pictures; souvenirs	

EXAMPLES FOR PRECISION TEACHING

Example Task 1: Verbs

- The therapist arranges about 10 picture or word cards with known actions (e.g., eating, swimming, driving) in a circle.
- The therapist sets the timer for 20 seconds.
- The therapist instructs the child to label as many cards as possible within a 20-second period.
- The therapist asks, "What is happening?," modeling the present progressive verb form.
- To start the trials, the therapist points to the cards in random order.
- Once the timer rings, the therapist records the number of correctly labeled verbs.
- For every increase in performance level, the child is praised and receives a token.
- Once the child exceeds his or her previous performance level three times, he or she receives a predetermined reinforcer.

Variations

- The targeted words are illustrated with different pictures.
- Learned actions are paired with a variety of subjects (e.g., the boy swims, the duck swims, the girl swims). Keep to singular subjects.
- At a later stage, the subject remains the same and the verb is changed (e.g., the horse runs, jumps, drinks).
- At a more advanced stage, the subject and verb are varied (e.g., I draw; the children play; the rabbit eats).

Notes

- The child should be able to recognize the label of the cards (hear–do), imitate the word (hear–say), and label it without model (see–say).

- Trainings of comprehension and expression can complement each other.
- The expected labeling rate of a competent speaker is 50 to 55 words per minute.

Example Task 2: Social Scripts

- Therapist and child look at a list of social situations that are either sketched or briefly described (see table of scripts below).
- The therapist sets the timer for 1 minute.
- The therapist asks the child to answer a set of listed questions as fast as possible.
- The therapist notes the correctness of the child's responses.
- The child is reinforced when his or her learning target has been met, which should be set at a higher level than the previous performance.

Prerequisites

- The child should be able to answer all questions on the list.
- The child should be able to use the selected scripts in everyday settings.
- The scripts should not be automatic or used spontaneously yet.

Note

The fluency standards for this exercise are unknown. Therefore, therapists should estimate fluency rate based on performance of typical peers.

The following table shows examples of frequently used social scripts. The child's responses are scored as positive if they are fast and appropriate.

What do you say when … ?

You	Response (+/−)	Someone	Response (+/−)	You _____ someone	Response (+/−)
are thirsty		needs help		run into	
are tired		asks, "How are you?"		meet	
are hungry		sneezes		recognize	
need a break		drops something		get to know	
need help		gives you a present		say good-bye to	
meet someone		makes you angry		want to help	

Note. + and − indicate correct and incorrect responses.

Form 7.28 shows how these examples could be recorded using the blank data form for precision teaching in Appendix 7.B.

Related Literature

Fabrizio, M. A., & Ferris, K. J. (2003). *Overview of fluency-based instruction for learners with autism.* Workshop at the CAABA, San Francisco.

Leach, D., Coyle, C. A., & Cole, P. G. (2003). Fluency in the classroom. In R. F. Waugh (Ed.), *On the forefront of educational psychology.* New York: Nova Science.

Form 7.28. Example data form for precision teaching of expanded communication.

Data Form for Precision Te

Child _____   Teacher _____

Skill Area   <u>Expanded Communication</u> _____

| Target Skill | Task Setup | | Time Unit | Consequence | Le H |
	Material or Task	Instruction			
<u>Actions:</u>					
Food and drink	"Cooking," "cutting"	"What is happening?"	Frequency in 20 seconds	Praise; token when performance im- proves from previous trial	S
Toys and games	"Catching," "building"				
Household	"Washing," "sweeping"				
School	"Working," "writing"				

EXAMPLES FOR NATURAL AND EXPERIENCE-BASED TEACHING

Example Task 1: Spontaneous Labeling of Objects

- Child and therapist take out groceries from a bag.
- The therapist hands the child a banana or other item and says, "We've taken out a banana."
- The therapist repeats the process with another banana, this time pausing between verb and object: "We've taken out a banana. There is another (pause) banana."
- If the child shows any communicative intent during the pause (e.g., eye contact, vocalization, imitation, spontaneous utterances), she or he is praised.
- Over the course of the session, increasingly more difficult communications are reinforced, such as past tense and category labels ("We bought a fruit").

Notes
- To make labeling easier, use objects bought in multiples (e.g., bananas, grapes, potatoes, wrapped candy). In the beginning of training, this gives children a better chance to succeed. Later, children can be expected to label a new item each time it is taken out of the bag.
- Sentence scripts should vary, such as, "Oh, another banana, and another," "So many grapes!" "Here is another grape, and some more."

Example Task 2: Reciprocal Communication

- The child and therapist or another child sit together with two similar objects before them (e.g., two hammers, two combs, two cars, two whistles).
- The therapist demonstrates an activity like blowing the whistle and says, "I have a whistle. I blow the whistle." "Show me the same."
- The child is praised when she or he imitates the activity.

- In the next step, the child is instructed to model the verbalization of "What are you doing?"
- Closer and closer approximations to the model are reinforced.
- In the last step, the language models are varied: "My car drives. Now it goes into a garage."

Variations
- The child is encouraged to follow his normal peers in play situations and to imitate utterances such as, "I eat," "I drink," "I buy."
- Scripted utterances can be practiced with binoculars ("I see"), taped sounds ("I hear"), or bags or boxes ("I feel").

Note
Figures 7.31 through 7.33 show various task setups that encourage reciprocal communication.

Table 7.6 provides examples of how natural teaching can be used to develop expanded communication skills. Form 7.29 shows a data form that can be used to record a child's responses to natural teaching. This form can be reproduced from Appendix 7.B.

EXAMPLES FOR VISUAL LEARNING

Example Task 1: Planning Future Events or Reporting Past Events

- The therapist interrupts the child who is about to start a liked activity, such as going for a bike ride, swimming, or playing, handing him a pictured activity schedule.

(text continues on p. 179)

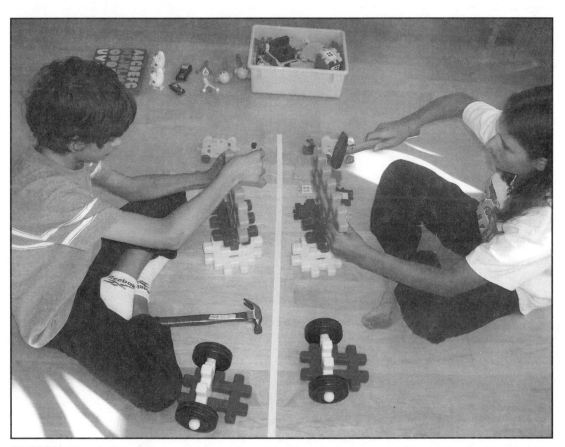

FIGURE 7.31. Two children doing activities together, such as hammering, can stimulate reciprocal communication.

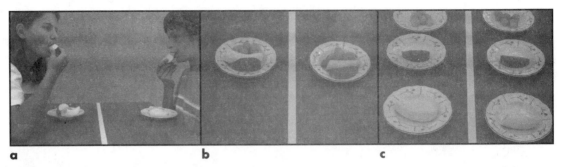

FIGURE 7.32. Reciprocal communication is encouraged by having children engage in various activities while sitting opposite each other at a table (a). Notice the clear boundary (i.e., white tape) in the middle (b). By changing the task setting slightly (c), children find it easier to communicate their differences in activities. Child 1: "I eat an apple." Child 2: "I also eat an apple." Child 1: "I eat some grapes." Child 2: "But I eat an apple."

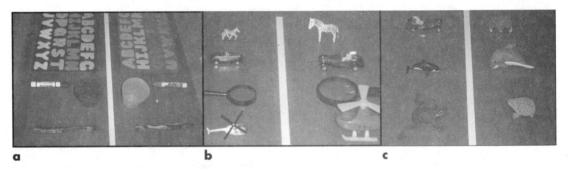

FIGURE 7.33. Reciprocal communication can be systematically practiced. Children can learn scripts such as the following: "I have a toothbrush." "Me too." (a). In another setting, they can talk about the size of their objects. One child has only small objects, while the other has only big objects: "I have a small magnifying glass." "I have a big magnifying glass" (b). Finally, this setup can help teach concepts such as the materials that objects are made of: "My frog is made of rubber." "My frog is made of wood" (c).

Form 7.29. Blank data form for natural and experience-based teaching of expanded communication.

Data Form for Natural and Experienc

Child _____   Teacher _____

Skill Area   Expanded Communication _____

Target Skill	Task Setup		Consequence
	Material or Task	**Instruction**	

Table 7.6
Examples of Ways Natural and Experience-Based Teaching Can Be Used To Develop Expanded Communication

Expanded Communication Skill	Examples Underline tested items
Spontaneity	Th: "This is a banana and another and another …"
Objects	Th: "What do you want?" "This is _____."
• Food	Ch: "Orange," "chocolate"
• Toys	Ch: "Ball," "Slinky"
• Household	Ch: "Refrigerator," "can opener"
• School	Ch: "Ruler," "eraser"
• Traffic	Ch: "Car," "bus"
• Utensils	Ch: "Saw," "screw"
Persons	Th: "Who (or what) is it?" "How does she feel?" "This shows _____."
• Relatives	Ch: "Aunt," "uncle," "cousin"
• Professions	Ch: "Bus driver," "secretary"
• Body parts	Ch: "Shoulder," "heel"
• Feelings	Ch: "Excited," "disappointed"
Living beings	Th: "What lives (or flies or swims) there?" "I see a _____." "Look, this is a _____."
• House animals	Ch: "Cat," "dog," "chicken"
• Zoo animals	Ch: "Lion," "monkey," "giraffe"
• Sea animals	Ch: "Dolphin," "whale"
• Birds	Ch: "Dove," "sparrow"
• Plants	Ch: "Tulip," "cactus"
• Trees	Ch: "Pine tree," "cherry tree"
Actions related to	Th: "What am I doing?" "What do you want to do now?"
• Food and drinks	Ch: "Cooking," "baking"
• Toys and games	Ch: "Building," "catching"
• Household	Ch: "Washing," "sweeping"
• School	Ch: "Working," "writing"
• Traffic	Ch: "Stopping," "directing"
• Utensils	Ch: "Stirring," "cutting"
Functions	
• Objects	Th: "What do you do with a radio (or sponge)?" "A radio is for _____."
• Body parts	Th: "What do you do with your ears?" "Ears are for _____."
• Locations	Th: "What are we going to do at the supermarket (or post office)?"

(continues)

Table 7.6. *(Continued)*

Expanded Communication Skill	Examples Underline tested items
Belonging	
• Objects	Th: "The CD belongs in the _____." Ch: "CD player"
• Locations	Th: (during play with a dollhouse) "Where shall we put the bathtub?" Ch: "In the bathroom."
• Categories	Th: "Where does the apple go?" Th: (while drawing) "Which animal can you put in the sky?"
Plurals	Th: "Eat a cookie (or some cookies)." "What did you just eat?"
Comparatives	Th: "What do you like the most (or least): baseball or tennis?" Ch: "I like baseball the most."
More-word utterances	Ch: "I see (or feel or smell) _____." Ch: "This is a _____." Ch: "I don't want _____."
Knowledge	
• Food and drinks	Th: "Where does the egg come from?"
• Vehicles	Th: "How many wheels does a car have?"
• Professions	Th: "Who brings the mail?"
• Animals	Th: "Which animals live in the pond?"
Calendar and time	Th: "How many days does a week have?" Th: "Which day comes after Friday?"
Time (adverbs)	Th: "Eat the cake first, and then drink the milk." "What did you do first?"
Prepositions	Th: "Where is the battery?" Ch: "Under (or behind) the pillow."
Pronouns	
• Personal	Th: "Who wants a cookie?" "Who has her lunch box?"
• Possessive	Th: "Whose watch (or shoe or ball) is this?" Ch: "Mine," "yours," "his."
• Demonstrative	Th: "Which game do you want to play?" Ch: "The one over there."
Questions	
• When?	Ch: "When are we going for a swim?"
• How?	Ch: "How can I open this?"
• Who?	Ch: "Who wants a dessert?"
• Which?	Ch: "In which box is my top?"
• Why?	Ch: "Why can't I go to the playground?"
Language functions	
• Greetings and farewells	Ch: "Hi," "hello," "good morning," "good night." Ch: "See you," "bye-bye," "take care."

(continues)

Table 7.6. (*Continued*)

Expanded Communication Skill	Examples Underline tested items
Language functions (*cont.*)	
• Instructions and orders	Ch: "Watch," "come," "join me," "leave me alone," "please get me a _____."
• Comments and interjections	Ch: "Okay," "agreed," "right," "no way," "but, really."
• Corrections	Ch: "No, it's not a _____," "I don't want _____," "I don't mean _____."
Reciprocal communication	Th: "I have a car." Ch: "I also have a car." Th: "My spoon is made out of metal." Ch: "My spoon is plastic." Ch: "I like Spiderman. How about you?"
Present, past, and future	Th: "What are you playing (or eating or watching)?" Th: "What did you just play (or eat or watch)?" Th: "What would you like to play (or eat or watch on TV)?"
Social scripts and compliments	Ch: "Thanks," "that's okay," "never mind," "I need a break." Ch: "That's a nice _____," "I like your _____," "well done!"
Conversation	
• Name	
• Age	
• Address	
• School	Ch: "What's your favorite class?"
• Family	
• Hobbies	
• Sports	Ch: "I like to watch basketball. Do you?"
• Television or computer	

Note. Th = therapist; Ch = child.

- The therapist asks, "What will you do now?"
- If the child does not reply, the therapist prompts a part of the action sequence (e.g., "Open the door," "Get my bike," "Take the helmet"), handing him the corresponding picture.
- Whenever the child responds with an appropriate approximation or comment, the therapist gives him access to that particular part of the activity sequence.
- If the child fails to respond, the therapist prompts either verbally or through pictures, word cards, or hand signs.

Variations
- The discussion of a picture sequence can be helpful in planning and verbalizing the different components of the action sequence.
- Putting the pictures of an action sequence into the correct order can also contribute to appropriate communication in the real setting.

Example Task 2: Social Scripts—"I Need a Break"

- Two therapists watch as the child is confronted with a frustrating task (e.g., assembling a puzzle with more pieces than usual).
- When the child shows signs of boredom or frustration, one of the therapists hands him or her the break card.
- The second therapist responds right away and gives the child a break.
- The timer is set for a specific amount of time (e.g., 3 minutes).
- Once the timer rings, all return to the task.

Variations

- As the child improves his or her ability to request a break, the second therapist is faded.
- Once the behavior is mastered, generalization to real-life settings is assessed.
- Scripts, such as one requesting a break, can also be trained using role-play or real-life settings.

Form 7.30 shows how these examples could be recorded using the blank data form for visual learning in Appendix 7.B.

Form 7.30. Example data form for visual learning method of teaching expanded communication skills.

Data Form for Visual Lear

Child _____   Teacher _____

Skill Area   Expanded Communication _____

Target Skill	Task	Instruction	
		Verbal	**Visual**
Past, present, future	"Eat," "ate," "will eat" "Play," "played," "will play" "Go," "went," "will go"	"What did you eat?" "What will you watch on TV?"	Picture, word, and hand sign sequence
Social scripts, compliments	"No," "yes," "thanks" "You are welcome" "Excuse me" "Is this vacant?" "I need a break"	"Do you need a break?" "I need a break"	Word card or hand sign

Play and Social Behavior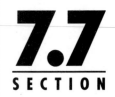

Section Overview

Importance of Play and Social Behavior

Questions for Evaluating a Child's Skills

Developmental Levels for Play and Social Behavior

How To Conduct the Training

Training Program Overview

Examples of Tasks for Developing Play and Social Behavior

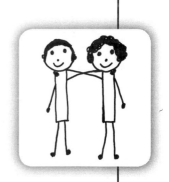

IMPORTANCE OF PLAY AND SOCIAL BEHAVIOR

Play, communication, and social behavior form an intricate relationship, with each area affecting the others. While playing, typical children learn important aspects of communicating and relating to others, such as having joint focus, taking turns, understanding consequences, imagining, sharing, negotiating, and many other communicative functions.

In children with ASD, deficits in play and social behavior often are the first indicators of atypical development. Many infants with ASD do not look at their parents and frequently are not aware of others. Their restricted perception is like tunnel vision, a perspective that includes only a small part of the world. They seem uninterested in toys and would rather engage in repetitive self-stimulatory activities such as spinning, waving, aligning objects, or jumping in place. While typical children learn, through imitation of movements and play, to focus on the interaction partner, children with ASD fail to share joint experiences, thereby missing many crucial learning opportunities (Quill, 2002). They often ignore their peers and get ignored in return. They are at risk of being rejected and excluded from group activities and are therefore denied the benefits of friendship.

Why are play and social behavior important?

- Understanding cause-and-effect relations
- Exploring one's environment
- Keeping oneself busy
- Perceiving others (through eye contact and joint attention)
- Taking turns and sharing with others
- Learning construction skills
- Building imagination
- Reacting to others' instructions and instructing others
- Communicating and coordinating views with others (e.g., requesting, describing, elaborating, clarifying, questioning)
- Considering the perspective of others (i.e., theory of mind)
- Learning about rules (e.g., behavior, games, hidden agendas)
- Understanding sayings, idioms, and jokes
- Taking on roles (e.g., mother, father, child; teacher, student; doctor, patient)
- Understanding and expressing feelings
- Developing empathy and friendship
- Giving and receiving help
- Giving and receiving compliments
- Giving and accepting constructive criticism
- Developing problem-solving strategies

Infants tend to explore the environment by mouthing, smelling, and feeling objects. They may engage in simple repetitive movement, such as touching a mobile or pushing a car back and forth. Through this *exploratory or functional play* they learn about the qualities and functions of objects long before these qualities get names, such as *hard* and *soft, heavy* and *light,* and even *plastic* and *cloth.*

An early experience of typical infants is discovering that their behavior affects the environment. When they touch a mobile, it moves; when they throw something out of their crib, it disappears. Positive consequences increase a behavior, while negative ones decrease it. If a mother repeatedly picks up a dropped object, the infant's throwing behavior is likely to occur more frequently. If, on the other hand, the mother scolds the infant, the throwing may decrease. During their first 18 months, infants engage in more and more reciprocal interaction with their caregivers by smiling, vocalizing, and looking at them, and infants are soon able to follow their caregivers' gaze (Berk, 1989). This taken-for-granted ability to follow another person's gaze is known as *joint attention*.

The development of joint attention is an important milestone because it forms the basis for communication and social behavior. Toddlers have to learn to take turns and share, which is often difficult because they consider themselves the center of the universe. Both behaviors— joint attention and turn taking—are important for later conversation as well as peer play, which should not be just egocentric entertainment, but satisfying to both parties.

While functional play can be observed in children before age 2 years, *pretend* and *constructive play* are the dominant play paradigms from the age 3 onward. A child may imagine that a block is a plane or that she or he is flying over the house. Some time later, children are able to take on roles, such as Spiderman, and instruct their playmates to take on other roles, such as firefighters. While playing, children learn to imagine, solve problems, explore concepts, improve their fine-motor skills, and even develop basic mathematical concepts.

Mike, 3 years old, is building a tower. He tries to find medium-sized wooden blocks and when he does, he places them carefully on top of each other. He calls his mother to show her his accomplishment. When his tower tumbles, he starts to collect all zoo animals. He discards the dog and the cow because he knows they are domestic, not zoo, animals. He builds a fence around the animals and searches for green plastic fence pieces. Because there is insufficient fence material, he closes the gap with a pencil. He announces his intent to build a cage and prepares the base by making a square of four long Lego bricks. He searches for the long red Lego bricks with 12 holes to build the bars of the cage. Because he is unable to find enough of them, he uses two Lego bricks with six holes each. After building the cage, he pretends that a truck comes with hay for the animals, and he makes loud munching sounds as he feeds them.

In the above example of a typical play situation, Mike practices a multitude of skills. Young children often talk to themselves, commenting on their play actions and sometimes even engaging in fictitious dialogue. In later stages of peer play, children use different forms of discourse, such as explaining, clarifying, questioning, sharing, negotiating, or asking for permission. They learn to take on different perspectives as they role-play. While playing, children find out who they enjoy playing with—and who they would rather avoid—thus forming the foundations of friendship.

Reduced Play and Play Level

Often, children with ASD follow their own restricted interests when playing. They may prefer self-stimulatory play, spinning any object that can be possibly rotated. They may collect all the Thomas the Tank Engines and create endless lines with certain objects. They may jump continuously on the bed or bore a listener with endless monologues about dinosaurs, birthdates, or other favorite topics. They often engage in these activities for extended time periods and seem oblivious to the world around them.

Many children with ASD must be directly instructed to play and to interact appropriately with others. They have to be taught how to take turns when playing ball, wait at the slide while another child has his or her turn, engage in a board game, or take part in role play. Without special help, they often play in isolation and therefore miss important steps in cognitive, motor, communicative, and social development.

Taking the Perspective of Others

Many children with ASD have difficulty seeing the world through other people's eyes or even recognizing their existence.

Mark, 4 years old, waves his hands in front of his eyes while walking to his favorite swing on the playground. He is unaware that he is walking directly into another child because he notices her only when it is too late to stop.

Ann-Marie, on the other hand, catches sight of a bag of chips in no time, but ignores the fact that a child is holding the bag. She seems surprised to be suddenly involved in a tug-of-war for her favorite snack.

Besides the above problem of "tunnel perspective," or being unable to perceive the presence of others, many children with ASD cannot put themselves into the shoes of other people to imagine how they must be feeling. They fail to understand that another person might not be able to see what they can see in the way that they see it.

When watching TV, Sue tends to sit right in front of her siblings, blocking their view. She cannot understand why they get angry because she cannot imagine that they cannot see the screen through her head.

Most people with ASD also have a hard time imagining that each person has different knowledge.

Coming home from school, 8-year-old Steven informs his mother that he was attacked by Bobby. Steven fails to mention, though, that Bobby is not a classmate but the neighbor's new dog.

Children, adolescents, and even adults with ASD have a hard time accepting that their behavior should "go with the flow." It is difficult for them to adapt flexibly to different people and different settings. They often are not aware that some things are mentioned only to certain people and in certain situations. Because they assume that everybody shares their perspective, they do not understand that people can be deceptive or will withhold, distort, or circumscribe information.

Coming down from the stage during the school concert, 11-year-old Larry announces loudly, "Now I really have to go pee." He ignores the fact that the audience laughs at his remark and that his classmates are embarrassed about the unfortunate end to their performance.

During recent years, the *theory of mind* concept (Baron-Cohen, Leslie, & Frith, 1985) has become key in autism research. Studies have demonstrated clearly that children with ASD cannot consider the thoughts, feelings, and beliefs of others.

One way that theory of mind has been tested is through the use of a picture sequence. The first picture shows two dolls named Sally and Anne, a marble, a basket, and a box (see Figure 7.34). In the next picture, Sally places the marble in the basket, then she leaves the room. Next, Anne plays a trick on Sally by moving the marble from the basket to the box. When asked where Sally will look for the marble when she returns, typical children correctly respond with "in the basket," while most children with ASD respond with "in the box." In this study, 80% of the children with ASD did not consider that Sally was not aware of the new location of the marble (Baron-Cohen et al., 1985).

Autism experts debate the relationship of lab-type tasks such as the above to the everyday problems of children with ASD and the impact of social-skills training on theory-of-mind

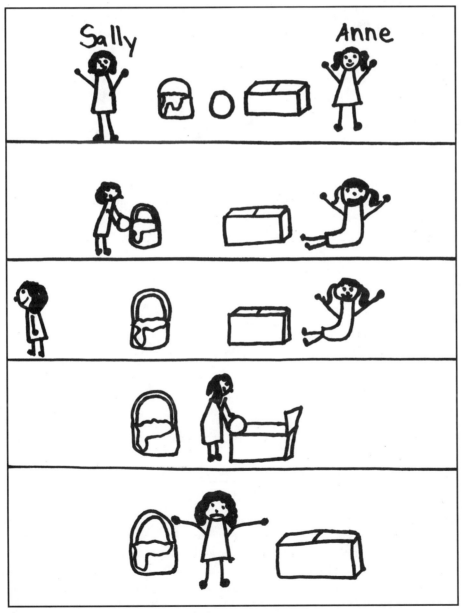

FIGURE 7.34. This series of pictures reveals whether a person has a theory of mind.

tests. In our research, high-level children with autism participated in social-skills training that focused on how to initiate a conversation, take turns during conversation, listen attentively, maintain a conversation topic, and change the topic appropriately. The children were tested on theory-of-mind tasks before and after training. Results showed that the amount of shared interest exhibited by the children with autism during conversation with their caregivers increased during training sessions. The children also made more responses that were appropriate to the context of the conversation. Performance on the theory-of-mind tasks, however, remained constant throughout the study (Chin & Bernard-Opitz, 2000), showing that an improvement in conversation skills might not necessarily demonstrate a change in theory-of-mind skills.

When To Say What to Whom and How

In social encounters, we normally consider the social context; unwritten rules about behavior; our knowledge, beliefs, and feelings; and the verbal and nonverbal communication of the interaction partner. For example, typical children communicate informally with their peers but speak deferentially to the principal. Students do not blurt out to the P.E. teacher that they detest P.E., and a student would reveal secrets to her best friend that her own brother would never hear.

Even elementary school children know that it is sometimes wise to hold back the truth to prevent trouble. When asked at night if he has brushed his teeth, a boy's confident "yes" does not reveal whether the teeth were brushed yesterday or today. White lies, excuses, and beating around the bush are rare in children with ASD. They usually are not good at small talk, but go straight to their topic of interest and give their opinion in a direct, honest way. A child learning not to speak her mind about the "bald man" at the checkout line, the "hair on the wart of the fat man," or the "big belly of the (pregnant) lady" would be an enormous relief for permanently embarrassed parents. Even the development of lying would suggest that a child has learned to take another person's perspective.

Knowing "when to say what to whom and how" is a continuous learning process for everyone, not only for those with ASD. We often have to judge within seconds whether our interaction partner agrees with us or whether continuing with our opinion may lead to frowning, ongoing tension, or even the start of close combat. This intricate adaptation to both the social setting and the interaction partner has to be made transparent for most people with ASD, and actually would be an eye-opener for many people without ASD. Being empathetic to others is not easy for either ASD or non-ASD people.

Considering the Feelings of Others

Even in everyday situations, people need a broad spectrum of sensitivity to the feelings of others.

A teacher who asks all her pupils to stand and then allows all those with an A grade to sit down first, followed by those with a B, then those with a C, and so forth does not seem aware of the desperation he is causing in the children with the lower grades.

Typically developing children who bully their peers through mobbing or physical attacks or who enjoy being cruel to animals are highly disturbed in their emotional development and empathetic response. This type of deviance is extremely rare in children with ASD and, when it does occur, often has different functions.

> Karen, a girl with autism, was fascinated by the tears of her baby sister and continuously checked where exactly they entered the eyes. To observe the tears, she sometimes even triggered the baby's unhappiness. She did not understand that tears are not just a mechanical process, but linked to certain experiences and feelings, such as thirst, hunger, pain, or discomfort.

Emotional intelligence (EQ) and communicative competence have been made popular by Goleman's (1996) bestseller *Emotional Intelligence* and related literature (e.g., Salisch, 2002). According to Goleman, human competencies like self-awareness, self-discipline, persistence, and empathy are of greater consequence in school, work, and private success than the intelligence quotient (IQ) and children should be taught these abilities. Because children with ASD are especially needy in this area, teaching EQ and social skills should be a major part of any training program.

Understanding Sayings and Abstract Language

Children, adolescents, and adults with ASD often think in a concrete way. They have obvious problems understanding abstract meaning such as that involved with well-known sayings. Remarks such as, "Zip your lips," "Shut up," or "Hold your tongue" are more likely to trigger pictures of zippers, lockers, and tongues, resulting in confused looks rather than the intended consequence of stopping the talk. Equally confusing are remarks such as the P.E. teacher shouting, "Do not run like lame ducks!" or the well-meant advice of a friend to "give the winning team the cold shoulder" (see Figure 7.35).

> A high-functioning child with autism, who had been integrated in his regular neighborhood school, called his former teacher of the autism class asking desperately, "I have to write an essay on a trip to the zoo. Why must we trip to the zoo?"

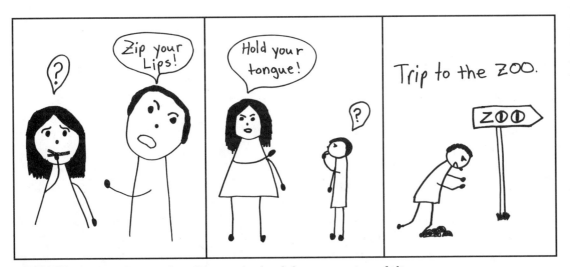

FIGURE 7.35. People with ASD often cannot comprehend abstract meanings of idioms.

Questions for Evaluating a Child's Skills

Play and social behavior are complex target areas that can be covered in this book only to a certain extent. Therapists should keep in mind that the previous sections on joint attention, language comprehension, and expressive communication are closely connected to this topic. More detailed programs can be found in the following references: Beyer and Gammeltoft, 2003; Howlin, Baron-Cohen, and Hadwin, 2002; McKinnon and Krempa, 2002; Quill, 2002; Schuler and Wolfberg, 2000; Winner, 2002; and Wolfberg, 2003.

The answers to the following questions are keys to understanding and helping children enhance their play and social behavior.

Questions to help determine the best way for a child to learn

- Does the child self-stimulate?
- If the child self-stimulates, is it predominantly visual, auditory, tactile, sensory, or vestibular (caused by the pleasure of movement)?
- Is the child able to play appropriately with different materials and toys?
- Does the child construct things?
- Does the child engage in imaginary play (e.g., pretending, role playing)?
- What is the child's preferred toy, game, hobby, or leisure activity?
- Is the child able to play alongside other children?
- Does the child participate in group games or activities (e.g., board games, recess games, music, cut-and-paste activities)?
- Who is available to play with the child (e.g., siblings, neighbors, classmates)?
- Is the child able to take turns with others?
- Is the child able to share toys and materials?
- Does the child play rule-governed games?
- Does the child understand sayings, jokes, and idioms?
- Is the child able to understand and express feelings and show empathy?
- Is the child able to consider the perspectives of others and put himself or herself into another person's situation?
- Is the child able to ask for and give help?
- Is the child able to understand hidden meanings and react accordingly?
- Does the child have friends?
- Is the child able to solve social problems?

Developmental Levels for Play and Social Behavior

Typical children make dramatic progress in play behavior during their first 5 years. They move quickly from isolated, exploratory play with their body, toys, or everyday objects to complex interaction and role-playing with others. During their second year, they engage in parallel play in which they observe and imitate the activities of others, comment on others' play, and find themselves interacting verbally and nonverbally. During the third year, they are able to take over small roles, such as pretending to be a fierce police officer, a frightened cat, or a roaring lion.

At this age they are able—though not always willing—to take turns. Cooperative play can be observed around the age of 4 years, where children follow simple rules such as in card, board, or outside games. At the age of 5 years, they can engage in complex role-playing and cooperative games (Johnson-Martin et al., 1990).

The social behavior of typical young children has an equally fascinating sequence of stages. As early as 3 to 6 months of age, infants smile back when someone smiles at them. At 6 to 12 months, they exhibit joint attention and are able to imitate the facial expression of the interaction partner. At 12 to 18 months, they exhibit clear interest in peers and react positively to the praise of adults. They offer toys and might be observed sharing or fighting over them. At the age of 18 to 24 months, they show off their accomplishments and take pride in their performance (Bayley, 1993; Weiss & Harris, 2001). At this tender age they already are able to comfort others. At the age of 3 years, they can label their feelings and have preferred friends. At the age of 4 years, they recognize when someone needs help and can offer help. One year later, at the age of 5 years, they usually have a group of friends.

This is typical development for most children. Children with ASD, on the other hand, need special instruction to develop the above play and social skills.

How To Conduct the Training

Unlike the previous sections, this one is not subdivided by different teaching methods (e.g., discrete trial format, precision teaching). Instead, the behavioral, developmental, and experience-based teaching methods are integrated in the training steps. At the same time, the questions most frequently asked by parents and teachers will be addressed:

How does my child learn to play?

- Isolated play

How does my child learn to play with other children?

- Parallel play
- Cooperative play
- Rule play
- Role play

How can my child learn to adapt better to various social settings?

- Integrated play groups
- Social skills groups
- Daily feedback
- Power cards
- Hidden curriculum
- Social stories
- Sayings and idioms

How does my child learn self-control?

- Problem bag
- Video feedback
- Self-evaluation
- Thought bubbles
- Behavior contracts

How Does My Child Learn To Play?

The development of play goes through different stages. It begins with isolated, sensory, cause–effect play and gradually moves through the stages of parallel play, cooperative play, rule-governed play, and, later, imaginary role play.

One of the first goals in developing play and social behavior in young children with ASD is the replacement of self-stimulatory play with functional and creative play. For young children, therapy is more likely to be successful if the toys and other materials used are close to perception channels or the children's interests.

Simon, 7 years old, waved any long object: a garden hose, twig, ruler, or even—to the embarrassment of its owner—an unfastened bikini top. In discussions with his parents, it was decided to take away the "wave objects" abruptly, saying, "no waving," and to replace them with similar visual toys. Appropriate play with these toys was reinforced by praise and small bits of food. Within 2 weeks, Simon's play behavior expanded significantly. Some time later, his self-stimulation was reduced to secret, unobtrusive twiddling of opened paper clips.

To obtain such speedy progress, therapists should conduct an analysis of the behavior problems and discover the child's interests and most frequently occurring activities. An important first question to answer might be: "Which perception channels are likely to be involved?" Table 7.7 lists alternatives to self-stimulatory play.

Children need to learn to play for extended time periods with a variety of toys or materials. Timers can be helpful for signaling how long a child can engage in a certain play pursuit. Pictured activity schedules can help a child move from one play activity to another, indicating, for example, that the child should first do the puzzle, then draw a house, and then put the bear to sleep.

How Does My Child Learn To Play with Other Children?

As a next step, children need to learn to play alongside other children in *parallel play*. To make them aware of their peers, toddlers can be placed in close vicinity of possible playmates, such as in playpens, in play corners, or on play carpets. Offering similar toys to both children also can enhance parallel play. Simple imitations of peers can be encouraged in such activities as building a tower and knocking it over, manipulating different switches of busy boxes, or activating noisemakers or battery-operated toys.

In small-group activities, children can be encouraged to develop an awareness of each other. Coordinating the movements of a parachute, hoops, or a big gymnastic ball can help a group of children find a common focus and observe peers, which promotes imitation and the sharing of emotions. Along with singing action songs, children can engage in joint drumming, tapping, rolling, stomping, or bouncing a gymnastic ball in the center of a circle. Language songs can link sung text to actions, objects, or people. There is no limit to what a creative therapist can do with this method.

Cooperative play involves children taking turns and participating in a common game (see Figure 7.36). Simple activities such as rolling a ball or pushing a car between two partners, taking turns building a tower, or inserting puzzle pieces can develop this skill. Small groups of children can connect cogs and wheels in such a way that turning one wheel activates the rest, thus reinforcing cooperative play via highly motivating spinning motions (see Figure 7.37).

Turn taking can be structured by letting the child whose turn it is wear a cap or hold a green *go* sign. A dividing line between two play partners with identical toys on both sides can

Table 7.7
Alternatives to Self-Stimulatory Behavior

Perception Channel	Self-Stimulation or Interest	Alternative Play
Visual	Waves objects	Jacob's ladder[a] Bead necklace Bubbles Balloons Lava lamp Torchlight (e.g., fiber-optic wand light) Flag (also unraveling flag) Slinky Parachute games
	Spins objects	Fan Pinwheel Tops with lights or sounds Tornado tops Linking wheels Fishing game (battery-operated) Cars or trains (with wheels of varying sizes) Helicopter Frisbee
	Aligns objects	Trains and tracks Magnetic cars or trains Stacking or nesting blocks and cups Duplo or Lego bricks Dominoes Jenga[b]
Auditory	Makes stereotypic sounds	Music or other distracting noise (e.g., water fountains, screen savers with sound) Musical instruments Headphones Noisemakers (e.g., rainmaker)
Tactile	Plays with water	Pouring water of different colors into containers of various sizes (or through funnels, filters, and sieves) Role-play such as preparing and serving tea
	Touching or feeling objects	Feely bag or box to guess objects by touching them Textured puzzles, letters, numbers, or dominoes Sand or water play Play-dough or baking dough Lotion Vibrating toys
Vestibular	Spins or twirls self	Hula hoop Circle games Swings Sit 'n Spin
	Jumps	Trampoline Pogo sticks

Note. For more information on the toys, see the following Web sites:
[a]http://www.woodcraftarts.com/jacob.htm
[b]http://www.hasbro.com/jenga

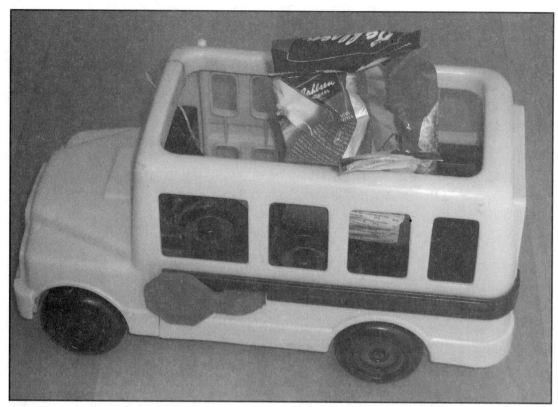

FIGURE 7.36. In this game that promotes cooperative play, children take turns pushing the bus to one another and taking a chip off the load upon arrival.

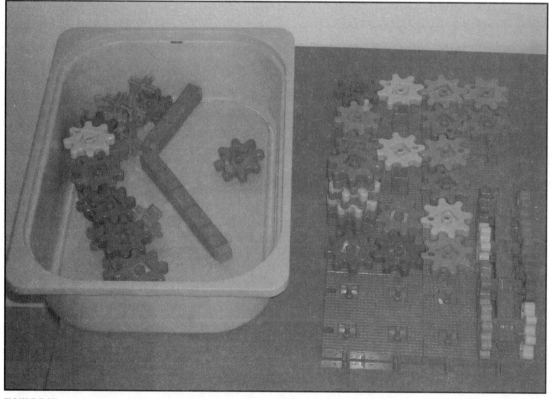

FIGURE 7.37. Taking turns is fun for children when favorite spinning activities are involved.

be a helpful visual prompt to facilitate turn taking as well as imitation and language (Beyer & Gammeltoft, 2003).

Many games can be split into various roles, so that one child blows bubbles while the others catch, smash, or poke them. With model trains, one child can set the trains on the tracks while the other activates the electric switch.

To move to the next play level, therapists should choose *rule-governed games* that are interesting for children with ASD. Children who love spinning motions are often highly motivated if they are allowed to catch plastic fish or ducks from a rotating disc. Card and board games can focus on the child's interest, be it numbers, letters, brand names of cars, or dinosaurs. Joining other children in tossing balloons or playing ball games, badminton, tennis, or table tennis creates superb opportunities for learning to cooperate and compete.

Role play can be considered the highest level of play development because it requires good imitation, expressiveness, and perspective-taking skills, and fantasy. To develop this level, therapists should focus play on certain topics, such as cooking, building, going to school, running a zoo or farm, or racing. In taking on the roles of farmers, teachers, and zookeepers, children learn to wait, share materials, follow and give instructions, expand their language, and communicate appropriately. By setting up various play stations in a room (see Figure 7.38), therapists can encourage children to follow their peers to the next activity. To prevent fixed play, therapists should vary play sequences daily and change materials weekly (Weiss & Harris, 2001).

For children with Asperger syndrome, play scenes can include special interests. Over the course of several sessions, the original interest can be varied and made more appropriate. Role playing a birthday party, for example, can be a good start for the child who is fascinated by birthdates.

Integrated playgroups offer good opportunities for siblings, peers, and children with ASD to learn from each other. Studies have shown that children with ASD who participate in integrated playgroups play more socially and less in isolation. They also play more functionally and less stereotypically with objects. Some of the children with ASD even demonstrated symbolic play in later sessions. In addition, advances in play behaviors were generalized to other contexts and were accompanied by language gains (Wolfberg & Schuler, 1993).

Research with 4- to 5-year-old children has demonstrated that typically developing peers at this early age can be good models for appropriate play. Children with ASD were observed imitating, without intervention from adults, the play activities of their typical peers (Carr & Darcy, 1990). Participation in the integrated playgroup produced dramatic increases in shared attention to objects, symbolic play, and verbal utterances, which continued even after the adult had left (McCracken & Wolfberg, 2005; Zercher, Hunt, Schuler, & Webster, 2001).

My colleagues and I also witnessed the development of play skills in our ASD children who participated in integrated playgroups, conducted once a week over a period of 10 sessions (Bernard-Opitz et al., 2004). The target behaviors in Table 7.8 were developed during a variety of activities.

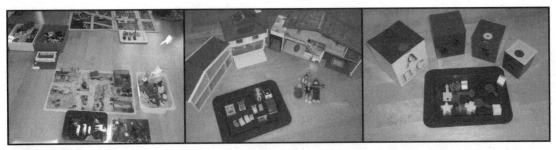

FIGURE 7.38. Play stations on specific topics and clearly laid out toys can help children with ASD to structure their play.

Table 7.8
Targets and Activities of Integrated Playgroups

Example of Social or Play Behavior	Target Behavior	Example of Play Activities
Cooperative play	• Joint attention • Imitation • Language • Shared emotions	• Parachute game • Circle game with language songs or musical instruments • Shadow or mirror games (with small and large movements such as nodding, hopping, or flying) • Simon Says • Bubble or balloon catching • Hula hoop train • Obstacle course (with tunnel, trampoline, beanbags)
Construction play	• Fine-motor skills • Joint attention • Imitation • Language • Sharing • Showing off	• Blocks or Lego bricks • Play-dough • Cardboard-house painting . • Tinkertoys
Rule-governed play	• Competition and cooperation • Speed • Numbers and time • Social awareness • Perspective taking • Shared emotions	• Magnetic or battery-operated fishing game • Card games • "Guess who" game • Musical chairs • "What's the time Mr. Wolf?"[a] • "Hit the pot"[b] • "Who is afraid of the big wolf?"[c]
Role-play	• Joint attention • Perspective-taking • Imitation • Language and social scripts • Expression of emotions	• Dress up • Parking garage or dollhouse • Restaurant, shop, or hospital • Zoo or farm • Birthday

Note. See the following Web sites for more information about these games:
[a]http://www.gameskidsplay.net/games/chasing_games/wolf.htm
[b]http://www.topics-mag.com/edition11/games-toddlers.htm
[c]http://www.gameskidsplay.net/games/chasing_games/wolf.htm

How Can My Child Learn To Adapt Better to Various Social Settings?

To behave appropriately, children—and adolescents and adults—have to attend to and interpret the social setting, adhering to social rules and expectations. Eye contact and joint attention are prerequisites for developing social skills (see first section of this chapter). While typical children acquire social behavior mainly by following others and without specific instruction, children with ASD have benefitted from STEP teaching to acquire these skills. The learning features of the child and his or her therapy targets must influence the choice of teaching method for it to be most beneficial.

Social Skills Groups

Social skills groups can help develop standard and individualized social skills in children with ASD. In such groups, participants learn various scripts for situations such as meeting someone new and giving and receiving compliments. In addition, the group can focus on individual social problems, which may have occurred in recent encounters. Group work can incorporate role-playing, and audio and video feedback, which are powerful tools for developing more appropriate social behavior (Weiss & Harris, 2001). Behaviors such as greeting someone with eye contact and other appropriate nonverbal behavior, taking turns, and entering a conversation are examples of skills that can be practiced in the safe environment of a social skills training group. Topics for role-play and video practice should vary from session to session and must include concrete examples of real-life encounters (McKinnon & Krempa, 2002; Shure, 2003).

Table 7.9 can be used to help participants in social skills groups evaluate videotapes of their behavior. It can also be used to assess generalization of learned behavior to everyday settings.

Daily Feedback

Some children with ASD like the idea of picturing a problem situation as videotape that they can rewind. Immediately after a problem occurs, they are asked to "wind the problem back" and to role-play a more appropriate way of behaving.

Christine, 12 years old, screamed and threw herself on the ground when her class listened to an outdoor street concert. Her therapist guided her to a quieter corner of the pedestrian mall and calmed her down. The therapist then demonstrated, through role-play, that Christine could ask for and listen to a portable CD player with headphones to block out the unwanted sounds of the concert instead of throwing a tantrum. Christine was prompted to practice the request a couple of times. After returning to the concert, she requested the CD player in the learned manner and listened to it.

Problem behavior can be discussed and modified in the real setting, but it also can be reflected on during daily feedback conversations at night. To make sure these bedtime sessions stay nonaversive, parents should use a "wind-the-day-back" strategy to focus on neutral and happy events in addition to the ones needing change.

Power Cards

For some children with ASD, picture cards of unwritten social rules have been helpful. These *power cards* are used to remind children of social rules during greetings, good-byes, sharing, or problem behavior (Gagnon, 2001). These cards provide a visual aid for developing appropriate behavior and can include a child's hero or special interests.

Table 7.9
Evaluating Videotaped Social Skills or Assessing Generalization

Setting	Eye Contact	Greeting	Waiting	Communicating
Playground				
Supermarket				
Bus				

Note. Indicate + or − for correct or incorrect behavior; NA if not applicable.

A hero such as Spiderman can become a friendly model who is able to face all of the conflict situations a child encounters. On an index card, Spiderman is pictured and the child is reminded of what to say and do in a particular situation (Weiss & Harris, 2001). Spiderman says the following when

- he bumps into someone: "I'm sorry" or "Excuse me"
- someone laughs: "What's so funny?"
- someone cries: "What happened?"
- someone attacks: "Leave me alone" or "Let go"

Hidden Curriculum

Children with ASD often fail in social settings because they are not aware of subtle behavior differences in different settings and with different interaction partners. While it may be acceptable for the child to talk about the "need to pee" or "change the pad" at home, it may be unacceptable to mention this in class or at a formal dinner. A concept called the *hidden curriculum* attempts to make explicit these differences in behaving, using methods such as direct instruction, cartoons, or power cards (Myles & Schapman, 2004). Even having social rules written on index cards and available in the real setting can be useful reminders, such as the following:

- "I only speak up in class when the teacher calls on me or I know the answer."
- "I do not talk about private needs to strangers or a group (toilet, sex, menstruation, sweating)."
- "When I get angry, I walk away and take 10 deep breaths."

Social Stories

People with ASD often experience social settings in ways different from those of people without this disability. Gray's *social stories* (2004) attempt to communicate social information in a clear and supportive manner. In comparison to the rule cards listed earlier, social stories do not strive directly for behavior change. Their main aim is to show the person with ASD the reasons for his or her frustration. At least 50% of the story should be directed at positive behavior and the previous efforts or successes of the child. This helps prevent the child's tendency to engage in catastrophic thinking. Stories are phrased in the first or third person, consist of 2 to 12 short sentences, and have a clear structure. In the introduction, the topic is described: a setting, an interaction, a concept, or a skill. In the middle, the hidden rules that have not been noticed by the child are made explicit. At the end, a conclusion is drawn (Gray, 2004). For some children, visualization through cartoons, photos, drawings (including the child's own drawings), or computer programs is useful (see Figure 7.39).

Examples of Social Stories

- Sometimes I don't get what I want. This makes me angry. When I am angry I can count to 10. If I manage not to get angry, my parents will be proud of me.
- When I lose something, I can ask someone for help to find it. My parents can help me search. We can think and search together.
- Sometimes I have to share my toys. When I share with others, they will share their toys. We can share our toys and have fun (Gray, 2004; Nah, 2000; Weiss & Harris, 2001).

Sayings and Idioms

Pictures of sayings and idioms and their abstract meaning can be helpful in making children with ASD, their peers, and other interaction partners aware that concrete and visual think-

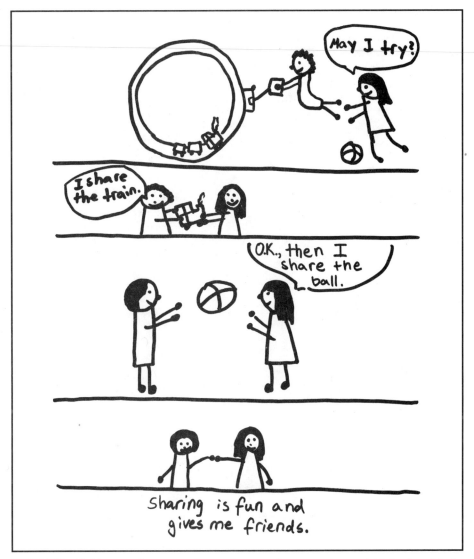

FIGURE 7.39. Children can learn to understand reasons for appropriate social behavior with the aid of social stories.

ing can lead to misunderstandings. Sensitizing teachers, parents, and peers to abstract language can be an important way of helping the integration of children with ASD. Table 7.10 gives examples of sayings and idioms that may be misunderstood by children with ASD and also provides a way to record the deliberate training of these phrases.

How Does My Child Learn Self-Control?

Visualization can help children with ASD develop self-control. In the social training groups organized by my colleagues and me, a picture of a *problem bag* was used as a starter. Group members were asked to write their problems on the picture of the bag and draw arrows to indicate which problems they wanted to tackle (see Figure 7.40). Evaluating one's own behavior as appropriate or inappropriate through audio and video feedback also is a valuable method of self-control. Audio or video samples of the child's appropriate and inappropriate tone of voice, posture, or other target behaviors are recorded, then the child listens or watches and scores each 10-second sample as *appropriate* or *inappropriate* on a checklist.

Table 7.10
Overview of Easily Misunderstood Sayings and Idioms

Saying or Idiom	Comprehension		Training Dates	
	Yes	No	Started	Ended
"Cool"				
"So long"				
"See you"				
"Let's hang out"				
"Zip your mouth"				
"Hold your tongue"				
"Shut up"				
"Hang in there"				
"I have a deadline"				
"He drives me crazy"				
"I'm fed up"				
"It's way above me"				
"Draw a conclusion"				
"Mind your own business"				
"Get fired"				
"Sleep tight"				
"Skip a line"				
"Hit a home run"				
"I have a frog in my throat"				
"Save your breath"				
"In the red"				
"I have cold feet"				
"He is the chair"				
"It's a lot of red tape"				
"Beat about the bush"				
"Bite off more than you can chew"				
"In a nutshell"				
"On the dot"				

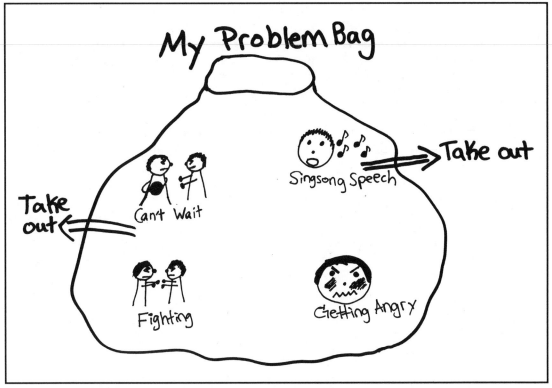

FIGURE 7.40. This exercise helps children with ASD tackle their social deficits through visualization.

"Do I speak normally or too high?" was the question 15-year-old Susan asked whenever she stopped the tape of her voice recording. The therapist praised Susan for her correct self-evaluations, even those that had an abnormal voice quality. Over the course of training, Susan became more and more aware of her voice and learned to speak in a more normal tone.

Training programs for self-control also can aim to improve the problem-solving skills of children with ASD. In a program developed by Camp and Bash (1981), children learn to brainstorm about possible solutions to a problem, select the best alternative, and evaluate their action plan. A picture of a bear planning to build a birdhouse is used to exemplify self-evaluation when problem solving. The bear asks himself the following:

1. What is the problem?
2. How can I solve it?
3. What plan is best?
4. Am I following my plan?
5. Did my plan work?

After several periods of training to make this self-evaluation in problem solving automatic, the child can tackle his or her current problems. Important components of this method are the following:

- A clear description of the problem (e.g., "My voice is too high")
- A clear goal (e.g., "I no longer want to speak in an abnormal voice")

- Alternative solutions (e.g., "I can practice a normal voice with my teddy bear, an audio-tape, or my Mickey Mouse doll")
- Choice of the best possible alternative (e.g., "I can practice with the audiotape")
- Tracking of progress (e.g., baseline: 10% of the trials are in a normal voice; after program: 60% of the trials are in a normal voice)
- Self-reinforcement (e.g., "I changed my voice and now I will call my old friend")

Thought bubbles, such as those seen in comic strips, can help children with ASD understand thoughts, beliefs, and false assumptions of other people. Children write their thoughts into drawn bubbles.

Thought Bubbles

Tim wishes for a rabbit (see Figure 7.41).
He thinks he will get a rabbit as a present.
He actually gets a scooter.
How does he feel?

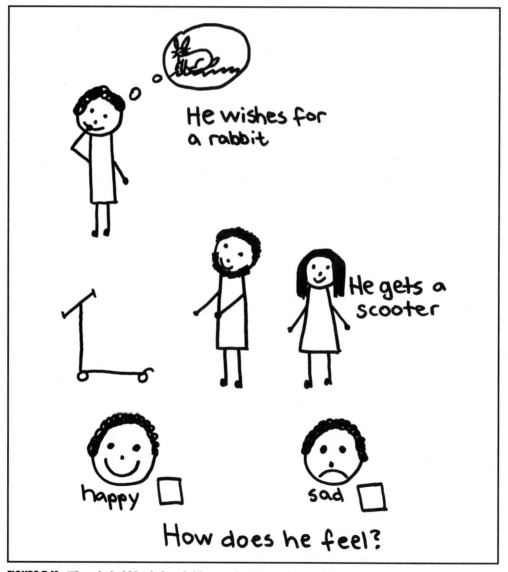

FIGURE 7.41. Thought bubbles helps children with ASD understand thoughts, beliefs, and assumptions.

Programs like thought bubbles have been shown to help children with ASD understand that other people have thoughts different from theirs (Howlin et al., 2002; Wellman et al., 2002). It has been demonstrated that autistic children of a mental age as low as 3 years understand that thought bubbles represent thoughts and that thoughts can be false. These results indicate that autistic children with a relatively low verbal mental age may be capable of understanding mental representations with visual support (Kerr & Durkin, 2004).

Children with ASD also can learn through role-play to discriminate between reality and pretend as indicated in the following example.

A boy with autism, Jacob, watches his sister Jane dress up as a dog, barking and crawling around the room. Jacob is asked if this is really a dog, if the dog really barks, and if it really has a tail. If necessary, Jacob is prompted to reply, "Jane is just pretending to be a dog" (see Figure 7.42).

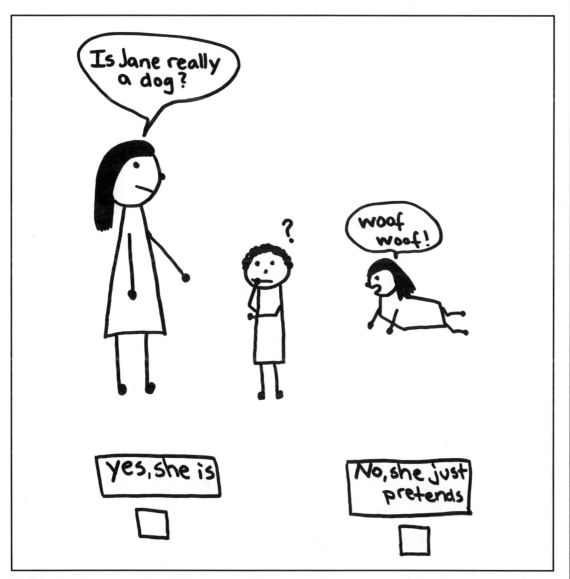

FIGURE 7.42. Role-playing helps children with ASD discriminate between pretend and reality.

To instill critical and less-naive thinking in children with ASD, therapists can have children role-play unlikely events. When an assistant enters the class insisting that he has just arrived from Mars or that he has found a golden treasure chest in the sandpit or that there is a horse flying over the roof of the school, the therapist can model how to handle unlikely reports. "Can this be true?" "Does it sound likely?" "Shall we really believe this?" Through role-play, children can learn to discriminate factual and fictitious information (Weiss & Harris, 2001).

Behavior contracts are another option for letting children with ASD share the responsibility for behavior changes (see Figure 7.43). The official look of the contract, the clear agreement about behaviors and consequences, and the confirming signatures can persuade children not to engage in emotional upheavals again and again.

TRAINING PROGRAM OVERVIEW

Form 7.31 outlines training programs to develop play and social behavior skills. The listed teaching targets should be assessed prior to the intervention and following a period of training. Once the child's profile of skills, learning channels, and interests has been determined, the therapist can select one of the four subsequent teaching methods. A reproducible copy of the form can be found in Appendix 7.A.

Contract

I _____ herewith promise my parents _____,
    (Name of the child)   (Name of the parents)

that starting on Monday, _____, I will call them when I am going to
                                (Date)

be more than 10 minutes late reaching home.

We, _____ and _____, promise that we will
    (Name of the mother)   (Name of the father)

let our son play an extra hour on the computer if he fulfills his contract.

_____

Child's signature

_____

Mother's signature

_____

Father's signature

FIGURE 7.43. Example of a behavior contract for arriving on time.

Form 7.31. Overview of the STEP training programs for play and social behavior; can be used as a pretest and posttest.

STEP Training Overview:
Play and Social Behavior

Child _____ Teacher _____

❐ Pretest ❐ Posttest

Play and Social Behavior Skills	Task Examples	Date Tested	Child's Response		Notes
			+	−	
Appropriate isolated play	Plays appropriately with:				
Sensory play	• Bubbles, tops, sand, and water toys				
Cause–effect play	• Jack-in-the-box, wind-up toys, busy boxes				
Construction play	• Duplo or Lego bricks, marble run, play-dough				
Imaginary play	• Vehicles, animals, people figures, dolls				
Parallel play	Plays parallel to another child for at least 10 minutes				

EXAMPLES OF TASKS FOR DEVELOPING PLAY AND SOCIAL BEHAVIOR

Example Task 1: Development of Turn Taking

- A child with ASD and his sister (or brother or peer) sit opposite each other on the floor at a distance of about 4 feet.
- The sister has a loadable vehicle (e.g., school bus, dump truck).
- The therapist hands the sister a toy or food items liked by the child with ASD, such as a raisin or flashlight.
- The sister is prompted to load the bus with the item and to get her brother's attention.
- Once the brother looks at his sister or the vehicle, she pushes it toward him.
- He is allowed to take the reinforcer from the vehicle and eat or play with it.
- The brother is prompted to push the vehicle back to his sister.
- The game is repeated about 10 times.
- Both children are reinforced for cooperative play.

Variations
- During the course of the training, the frequency of the material reinforcement can be reduced to about every third or fifth time the bus is exchanged.
- The distance between the children can be increased over the trials.
- Rolling objects such as balls, marbles, bottles, and cans can be used.

Example Task 2: Considering the Perspectives of Others

- A child with ASD pretends to be a waiter in a restaurant.

- The child asks the "guests" (i.e., peers) what drinks they would like to order.
- The child repeats their orders to the "waitress," another child who serves the drinks.
- The child brings the ordered items to the guests.
- Whenever the child makes mistakes, such as ordering and delivering her or his own favorite drink instead of the wanted item, she or he is corrected.
- At the end of the role-play, the child is allowed to order her or his own favorite drink.

Variations

- The list of the guests' orders can get increasingly longer over the game. Besides drinks, food items, snacks, and desserts can be added.
- The distance from the guest tables to the bar can become increasingly longer.
- Distractions can be introduced between getting the order and passing it on.

Example Task 3: Offering and Giving Help

- An assistant of the therapist loads more books, magazines, or toys in his arms than he can carry.
- When opening the door, some items drop.
- The child is alerted to the assistant's mishap and is prompted to ask, "Can I help?" (see Figure 7.44).
- The child is reinforced for repeating the phrase and helping.
- The procedure is repeated at other doors.

Variation

Other situations requiring assistance are role-played, such as the following:

- A handle rips off a paper bag that is too heavy.

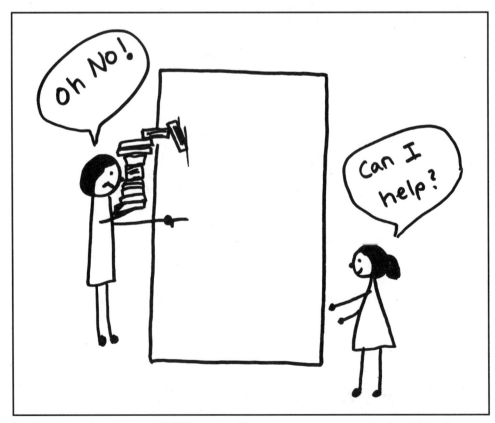

FIGURE 7.44. In this exercise, a child learns to offer assistance to someone who has dropped an item.

- A smaller child tries in vain to put an oversized battery into a toy.
- Someone pretends not to know how to turn on the computer, TV, or radio.

Example Task 4: Giving and Receiving Compliments

- In a social training or integrated playgroup, children sit in a circle and are asked to take turns, going clockwise, giving each other compliments. They are to comment on external features such as clothing or hair.
- After the first round of compliments, children are asked to say, "Thank you" after each compliment on the next round.
- Once children have mastered this exchange, they are requested to return compliments.
- In the last step, children expand the topic by adding details about the mentioned positive feature, such as, "Thanks! I used a new shampoo for my hair." "Thank you. My grandma gave me the T-shirt."
- The children are praised for successful performance.

Variations
- Once the children have mastered commenting on external features, they can practice making positive comments on personal features, skills, hobbies, and interests.
- The game can be played with a timer to help children become more automatic in saying positive things to each other.

Related Literature

Beyer, J., & Gammeltoft, L. (2003). *Autism and play.* London: Kingsley.

McKinnon, K., & Krempa, J. (2002). *Social skills solutions: A hands-on manual for teaching social skills for children with autism.* New York: DRL Books.

Schuler, A. L., & Wolfberg, P. (2000). Promoting peer play and socialization: The art of scaffolding. In A. Wetherby & B. M. Prizant (Eds.), *Transactional foundations of language intervention.* Baltimore: Brookes.

Weiss, M. J., & Harris, S. L. (2001). *Reaching out, joining in: Teaching social skills to young children with autism.* Bethesda, MD: Woodbine House.

Self-Help Skills and Independence

Section Overview

Importance of Self-Help Skills and Independence

Questions for Evaluating a Child's Skills

Developmental Levels for Self-Help Skills and Independence

How To Conduct the Training

Training Program Overview

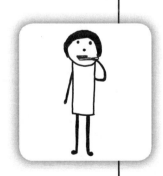

IMPORTANCE OF SELF-HELP SKILLS AND INDEPENDENCE

Parents, teachers, and therapists usually are quite concerned when a child's self-help skills and independence do not develop at the expected age. This is true for children of all ages. A child with ASD who is not toilet trained is not always welcome in regular preschools and might be even less accepted by his peers in an elementary school. An adolescent who is academically capable, but fails to dress himself and still needs supervision for basic personal hygiene, is also considered a problem. Typical peers can be quite outspoken when their classmate repeatedly forgets to check his zipper after a visit to the toilet or fails to get the shampoo out of his hair after a swimming lesson.

Why are tasks for self-help skills and independence important?

- Age-appropriate development
- Personal independence
- Positive self-concept (e.g., "I can do it on my own")
- Prerequisite for preschool
- Integration with typical peers
- Relief for parents, teachers, and others

For many adolescents and adults with ASD, their dependence on others is highly restricting. They often require extensive assistance in maintaining personal hygiene, such as dressing and undressing, or finding the cafeteria at school. Problems with organization interfere with school and professional success.

QUESTIONS FOR EVALUATING A CHILD'S SKILLS

To get a better picture of a child's level of independence, therapists can use instruments that assess daily living skills (Johnson-Martin et al., 1990; Sparrow et al., 1984). In addition, parents, teachers, and other relevant informants can be interviewed about problem areas that go beyond standard checklists. For example, a question like, "Can your child use public bathrooms or is she afraid of a noisy hand dryer?" might reveal a problem that limits a family's willingness to go on outings with their autistic daughter. "Is your child able to select an appropriate urinal and behave safely in a men's bathroom?" may be a pertinent question for a family with an older autistic boy. In both cases, the social context and the parents' priorities for teaching targets are important for ensuring that learned skills are generalized to the child's environment. For example, a therapist's efforts to teach shoe tying may be futile and a waste of valuable time for a child who wears tennis shoes with Velcro straps like the rest of her family.

Furthermore, the instruction "Describe a typical day from morning to evening" often provides important additional information to the questions asked on interview scales. The answers to the following questions will provide information about a child's current level of functioning.

- Which activities of daily living can the child do independently?
- Where does the child need help?
- Is the child able to wash herself or himself and shower independently?
- Can the child brush her or his teeth independently?
- Can the child comb hair and dress herself or himself independently?

- Is the child able to do and undo buttons, zippers, and shoelaces?
- Is the child toilet trained during the day and at night?
- Is the child able to pour juice and make a sandwich?
- Is the child able to eat with a knife and a fork (or chopsticks, for an Asian child)?
- Is the child able to help with household chores, such as making the bed, storing toys, or fixing simple meals?
- Can the child move around the neighborhood unsupervised (e.g., to visit friends, to ride a bicycle to school, to go shopping)?

While the above questions are related to the child's age and developmental level, the child's cultural background and practices, as well as the parents' value system, will determine whether making a sandwich, for instance, is more important than learning to eat with chopsticks. To plan appropriate intervention, the following key questions should be asked:

Questions that help determine the best way for a child to learn

- Are deficits mainly due to a lack of skills or a lack of motivation?
- Are fine-motor problems interfering with dressing, eating, and so forth?
- Is the child able to sequence simple actions?
- Is the child able to imitate?
- Does the child respond better to language, pictures, word cards, or hand signs?
- Which situations provide good incentives for learning self-help skills?
- Is the child dependent on prompts?
- Is the child able to structure her or his day independently?
- What are powerful incentives for the child?

In addition to determining parents' priorities, it is important to determine the prerequisites a child needs to be able to reach certain goals. For example, does the child have the necessary fine-motor skills to finger-feed or eat with a spoon, knife, and fork? Is the child able to comply with verbal commands, imitate motor movements, or follow pictured schedules indicating where exactly to brush his or her teeth?

To develop independence, children must learn a variety of activity sequences. At an early stage they need to know that going outside, for example, requires at least three steps: putting on socks, putting on shoes, then opening the door and going outside. At a later stage, children need to learn more complex sequences, such as the 10 or more steps involved in washing hands, tying a shoelace, or making a simple meal.

The third key question involves motivational issues. Is the child more motivated to learn through natural consequences (e.g., jumping into the pool after changing independently into swim trunks) or external incentives (e.g., receiving a goodie for changing the hamster's bedding)? Should the self-help training be embedded into everyday activities at home or practiced in a separate session? With which person and in which setting does the child perform best? The answers to these questions will help guide the child's training program.

DEVELOPMENTAL LEVELS FOR SELF-HELP SKILLS AND INDEPENDENCE

Developmental milestones in fine-motor skills and cognitive and language development serve as an important basis for self-help skills and independence. When a child searches for a tissue in Mom's purse to blow her nose, or scissors to cut a hurting cuticle, he or she is remembering that objects out of sight still exist. This skill, called *object constancy,* normally develops between the ages of 6 and 9 months.

In typical infants, the development of fine-motor skills, such as grasping and releasing at around ages 4 to 5 months, constitutes a big step toward independence (Bayley, 1993). At around age 7 months, they can hold their own bottles. At the age of 9 months, they are able to pick up objects with a pincer grasp and release them. At around age 12 months, they are able to finger-feed. One year later, they can eat with a spoon and drink from a cup they hold themselves. At age 3, they can prepare a bowl of cereal with milk, and 2 years later, they can spread butter or peanut butter on bread (Johnson-Martin et al., 1990).

Children as young as 12 months are very happy to take their socks and shoes off, but putting them back on remains the parents' job until children are about 30 months old. Only at the age of 3 years are they able to handle different fasteners. Buttoning is one of the more difficult skills, developed at age 4 years. At the age of 5, children are able to fully manage the zipper of their jacket or coat.

Small children usually enjoy water play, so they will cooperate with hand washing. This starts at around the age of 15 months, but only by the age of 3 years are they able to wash their hands independently. Brushing teeth independently is a more difficult task involving a sequence of several steps, and this is not usually mastered until the age of 4.

Parents often are very eager for their children to be toilet trained, which tends to come all by itself around the age of 3. Most 5-year-olds, though, still require help with wiping themselves and may sometimes have accidents at night.

Other developmental accomplishments can be observed outside of the home environment. In areas with little traffic, 3- or 4-year-olds can be seen exploring the neighborhood alone riding their push cars or tricycles. Parents should remember, though, that safe behavior at traffic lights and crossings cannot be expected before entry into school. Most children will enjoy their first steps toward independent shopping, be it handing the money from Mom to the cashier, putting coins into a drink machine, or—at a later stage—buying something from the nearby grocery store without any adult assistance.

In comparison, children with ASD show clear deficits and abnormalities in various self-help skills. While one group of parents worries about the limited types of food their children eat, other parents may focus on sleep or toileting problems. Some parents of older children are concerned about their children's general lack of independence or problems in organizational skills.

How To Conduct the Training

Task analysis, behavior analysis, activity schedules, and self-management are core methods in the development of self-help skills and independence.

Task Analysis

To develop complex self-help skills, such as dressing or attending to personal hygiene, in children with ASD, therapists must create *task analyses.* Here, a target behavior, such as making a sandwich, is broken down into its component parts, one of which is spreading butter on the bread. While this step sounds rather simple, it is really quite complex: One has to get the correct amount of butter on the tip of the knife (without the butter falling off), turn the knife in such a way that the butter actually ends up on the bread, and then distribute more butter on the bread than on the table or one's hands. In addition, the way a sandwich is made may differ among families and cultural groups; it is useful to let parents describe or demonstrate tasks.

In addition, standard task analyses such as for brushing one's hair or making a phone call can be used to help find subskills (e.g., Baker et al., 2004), such as: Is the child able to bring the hairbrush to the different parts of his hair? Can the child dial a phone number and introduce herself? These can be pictured in photo sequences or schematic drawings, or described in words.

Usually tasks are trained in a *forward chain,* meaning that training starts with the first step and proceeds to the second step, and so forth. For example, to feed himself, a child first has to learn to pick up the spoon, then scoop up some food, and finally bring the spoon to his mouth. Sometimes reversing this order, called a *backward chain,* is more motivating. A child who gets help with the first steps of feeding and only has to complete the last step of putting the food into his mouth independently tends to be more motivated.

Marcel was frustrated when shown the complicated series of steps for tying shoes: (1) Grab the end of the shoelaces. (2) Pull them apart. (3) Cross them. (4) Make a loop, and so on. He tended to lose interest at the third step and would not participate in the rest of the activity. To motivate him, the therapist used a backward chain. To begin, all Marcel had to do was to complete the last step of the chain, pulling the finished bow tightly (the therapist had done the rest of the task). After that, he was immediately allowed to walk away. On the next occasion, Marcel did not mind doing the last *two* steps on his own, then the last *three* steps, and so on, until he had mastered the complete task.

Behavior Analysis

For children with behavior problems, therapists are advised to conduct a *behavior analysis* to help define the causes and functions of the behavior. Likewise, children's problems in self-help skills need to be understood before an intervention program is set up. There may be various reasons why a child is not learning certain self-help skills. Consider the following example of buttoning:

- If a child cannot button, one reason may be that she usually gets help and therefore does not have an opportunity to practice the task. Obviously, she should be provided with more occasions to rehearse this skill.
- Another reason may be a delay in the child's development of fine-motor skills. Such a child is likely to benefit from training in manual dexterity. Activities such as taking clothespins off the rim of a basket, box, or laundry line; pressing the trigger of water guns; kneading dough; polishing silverware; or peeling potatoes can strengthen a child's hand muscles.
- Still another reason a child may not have learned to button could be a lack of attention to the training. In such cases, my colleagues and I have been successful when using traditional reinforcers combined with unconventional exercises. Imagine how much fun it is to pass a gummy bear or an M&M through a buttonhole and then get to eat it!

A behavior analysis can reveal whether deficits or lack of interest is the cause of any failure to make progress. Sometimes the therapist must deal with a lack of skill first and a lack of motivation later.

Sara, 5 years old, used to tantrum and go limp when asked to change into her pajamas and go to bed. Whenever her mother took her swimming, however, Sara could not wait to undress, ripping her clothes off and practically jumping into her bathing suit.

The above example clearly shows that Sara's inability to undress was not due to problems with fine-motor skills or a lack of knowing which item to shed first. Instead, her problem likely was a lack of motivation to undress at night. The positive consequence of swimming was a sufficient incentive for Sara to change her attire. Based on this history, one could say that her behavior problem has a good chance of being modified by reinforcement of undressing. At night, Sara could be allowed to take a bath in the bathtub if she undressed independently, or could be promised a visit to the pool the following day. To help bridge the time gap between her positive behavior and the consequence, a picture sequence could be set up, such as the following: Sara undresses; she sleeps in her bed; she goes to the pool.

Juan-Carlos becomes quite frustrated because he cannot unzip his raincoat or untie his shoelaces. In this case, it may be advisable to let him practice handling zippers and laces in a table-type setting. Meanwhile, Velcro fasteners can be introduced in the real setting until he has improved his dressing skills.

Sometimes, parents and other responsible adults may consider it too strenuous and time-consuming to conduct self-help training. A vicious cycle in which the adult helps the child and the child becomes prompt dependent can develop, leading to a situation called "learned helplessness" (Seligman, 1975).

The mother of 7-year-old Cheryl complained that she still had to feed her daughter. A behavior analysis revealed that the child was fed so frequently that she was possibly not even experiencing the feeling of being hungry. To test if regular hunger pangs would make her eat by herself, Cheryl's "breakfast" was scheduled at lunchtime in our clinic. Cheryl's mother could not believe it when she witnessed through the one-way window that her daughter was quite able to eat by herself.

It is not always as easy as this to reduce or even to eliminate problems with eating. Often, a child's long history of insisting on a few specific food items can be highly resistant to change. However, the following steps have been effective even in difficult cases.

1. First, the therapist must assess whether the child shows the food preference across various settings and people and not only with the mother at home or the teacher in school. If certain people are a factor, then letting the mother sit in on the school snack or inviting the teacher to afternoon tea at home can help merge the child's incompatible worlds and reduce the problem.

2. A second option is to examine the specific characteristics of liked and disliked food. Many children with ASD do not like to chew hard food or experience certain textures. To reduce this oversensitivity, oral–motor stimulation or mesh chewing bags can be helpful (see Baby Safe Feeder, http://www.beyondplay.com). Experienced speech–language pathologists should be consulted in these cases. In addition, some children dislike certain types of food, such as vegetables, fruit, or meat, or certain food colors, such as green. Masking the disliked feature by mixing it in with liked food has often been successful. One example is hiding minced meat or vegetables in favorite dishes or providing vegetable drinks. Even unusual combinations such as Smarties sprinkled on the disliked carrot dish or meatballs decorated with chips can be attractive to children.

3. A third option is to reinforce eating of nonpreferred food items. This corresponds to Grandma's rule of first eating what you dislike, even just a tiny piece, quickly followed by eating what you do like.

Children who do not or cannot brush their teeth appropriately also have their reasons.

- One child may not have sufficient observation skills to note that Mom models brushing the lower back teeth and instead brushes the sides of his teeth.
- Another child may not brush her teeth because of problems imitating the movement.
- A third child may refuse to cooperate because of oversensitivity in his mouth.
- A fourth child may have problems with awareness of his body.
- Finally, a fifth child might find nothing more boring than toothbrushing!

Each individual case warrants a corresponding treatment. Imitation training or pictured mini-schedules could help the first two children, while desensitization training seems the right choice for the third child. This child also may be less reluctant if the toothpaste tastes like chewing gum or some other flavor. In some extreme cases where a child refuses to even open the mouth for the toothbrush, brushing the teeth with Nutella spread has helped make the activity more attractive. Obviously this should be conducted only as a short-term emergency intervention, and it requires plenty of rinsing to prevent it from doing more harm than good. Children such as the fourth child, who do not have a good perception of their various body parts, sometimes perform better with visual feedback such as brushing teeth in front of a mirror. As for the fifth child, the therapist or parent may find that relating the toothbrushing to a story, a favorite cartoon character, or a song might do the trick. See Figure 7.45 for another toothbrushing motivator.

Successful toilet training is another milestone in a child's independence, and it is usually not easy for children with ASD. Parents often struggle with their child's prolonged bed-wetting or -soiling. Some children withhold their urine or bowel movements, while others urinate too frequently. Once a medical assessment has ruled out possible physical causes, a behavior analysis can clarify whether cognitive or psychological reasons underlie the problem. Likely causes include propensity for compulsive behavior, demand avoidance, or desire for attention.

Children with severe disabilities often are not aware of their body functions, so they must become sensitized to their bladder and to know when to initiate proper toileting. In many cases the following intensive training has been successful.

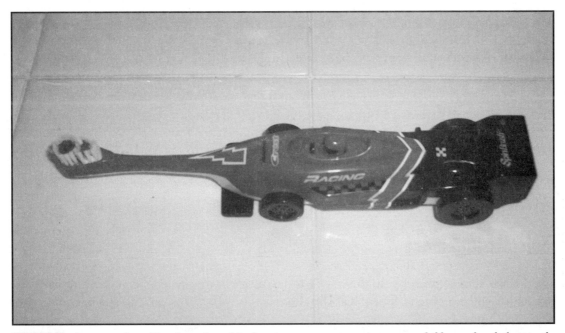

FIGURE 7.45. An unusual toothbrush, such as this electric race car, can motivate some children to brush their teeth.

- To trigger the need to go to the toilet, a child is prompted every half hour to drink as much as possible. Chips and other salty snacks can help make the child thirsty.
- Before his next drink, the child must sit on the toilet for 5 to 10 minutes.
- For successes on the toilet, the child is praised and receives a material reinforcement.
- If an accident occurs, the child is reprimanded and rushed to the toilet.
- After briefly sitting there, he is prompted to pull up his pants, wash hands, and return to the place where the accident happened.
- The last step is repeated several times to practice the correct behavior.

While children tend to dislike this overcorrection, the method has been found to be very successful (Azrin & Foxx, 1981; von Gontard, 2004).

For children older than age 6 years who have no medical reasons for wetting and none of the above behavioral reasons, bedwetting alarms have been successful. A wet-pants alarm is a small electronic device that makes a sound or vibrates when the child urinates in her pants. These alarms can be used for day or night wetting.

The use of overcorrection in conjunction with the alarm systems often causes marked progress within 1 week. Because both methods are aversive interventions, they should be discussed with all involved parties and supervised by experienced behavior therapists.

Activity Schedules

An activity schedule is a set of pictures or written words that encourages someone to perform an activity (McClannahan & Krantz, 1999). Comparable to a list of daily chores, an activity schedule serves as a reminder of what to do. Because children with ASD often have problems imagining upcoming events and organizing their behavior, activity schedules have proven extremely helpful. Unexpected changes in routine schedules often cause children with ASD severe distress, but announcing the change in their planners ahead of time can alleviate the problem. Autistic children as young as 3 years old can learn to follow their pictured schedule and move without adult supervision from one activity to the next. In the beginning, a simple picture schedule at home may cue a child to get up, go to the bathroom, and then eat breakfast. At a more advanced stage, a pictured or written schedule may help the child in preschool with the transitions from the morning circle to individual therapy to group session to snack time.

Mini-Schedules

Mini-schedules can help a child visualize details of an activity. "What exactly is expected of me in the bathroom?" "How can I fix my own breakfast?" "How do I make pizza?" A pictured or written sequence may aim at either general activities, such as "Toileting," "Washing," "Brushing teeth," or "Combing hair," or at specific steps, such as, "Go to the toilet," "Pull down pants," "Sit down," and so forth. (For further details, see Abrams & Henriques, 2004; Hodgdon, 2000; McClannahan & Krantz, 1999).

Self-Management

To develop self-sufficiency, children need to learn to become independent of others. Simple checklists with specific tasks, such as the chore list in Table 7.11, can help them monitor their accomplishments.

Table 7.11

Example of Self-Management List for Chores

Daily Chores	Done
Make my bed	
Set the table	
Feed the fish	
Empty the trash	
Rake the leaves	

TRAINING PROGRAM OVERVIEW

Form 7.32 summarizes important self-help tasks and exemplifies teaching strategies. Because of the vast scope of this topic and limited space, the task examples are brief and are not labeled by teaching method. The reader is referred to specialized readings such as Baker et al. (2004). A reproducible copy of the form can be found in Appendix 7.A.

Example Task 1: Brushing Teeth

Step 1
- The therapist stands behind the child at the sink and says the following: "Let's brush our teeth. Show me your teeth."
- If the child responds, he or she is praised.
- If the child does not respond, the therapist points to his or her own teeth and praises the child for modeling.
- The therapist brushes the child's front teeth and her or his left side in a gentle circular movement while saying, "Up and down, up and down."
- The therapist takes the brush out, turns his wrist, and brushes the right side and makes the same comment.
- The therapist asks the child to rinse his mouth with a sip of water.
- If necessary, the therapist demonstrates spitting out the water.
- The therapist brushes the biting surfaces of the teeth in the same order while saying, "Back and forth, back and forth."
- The child gets another sip of water for rinsing and is praised for brushing his or her teeth.

Step 2
- In subsequent sessions, the therapist guides the child's hand.
- The therapist interrupts the movements to see if the child continues on the therapist's verbal comment.
- If the child continues the movements alone, he or she is praised.

Step 3
- As the child makes progress, the therapist fades his or her physical guidance further, touching only the child's elbow and later only pointing to the teeth and commenting.

Form 7.32. Overview of the STEP training programs for self-help skills and independence; can be used as a pretest and posttest.

STEP Training Overview:
Self-Help Skills and Independence

Child _____ Teacher _____

☐ Pretest   ☐ Posttest

Self-Help Skills	Task Examples	Date Tested	Child's Response +	Child's Response −	Notes
Meals and snacks					
• Eating	• Eats small pieces of food by hand • Eats a snack or meal by hand • Eats with spoon • Eats with knife and fork				
• Drinking	• Drinks from a training cup • Drinks from a regular cup				
• Sandwich making	• Spreads butter on bread • Adds meat, cheese bread in half				

- Once the child is independent in brushing his or her teeth, he or she is prompted to complete the whole toothbrushing sequence: Turn on water, fill cup with water, open toothpaste, put toothpaste on the toothbrush, close toothpaste, brush teeth, rinse, clean sink, put toothbrush away, and clean up afterward by himself or herself.

Variation

Some children respond well when counting or timing is added:

- The comments "up and down" and "back and forth" can be replaced by rhythmic counting: "One, two, three, four, five, and ... One, two, three, four ..."
- Action songs on toothbrushing can be added (e.g., "This is the way we brush our teeth ...").
- Visual and auditory timers can be used to give the child feedback over the required duration of the activity.

Note. Steps 1 through 3 adapted from *Steps to Independence: Teaching Everyday Skills to Children with Special Needs*, by B. L. Baker et al., 2004, Baltimore: Brookes.

Example Task 2: Helping Around the House

- The child has a list of pictured or written household chores, such as making her or his bed, setting the table, cleaning her or his room, and sorting the laundry.
- To the right of each item on the list is a box for checking off completed tasks.
- At the bottom of the page is a picture of a reinforcer.
- The child works from the top to the bottom of the list.
- After the child finishes a task, she or he checks the appropriate box.
- Once all jobs are done, the child gives herself or himself the pictured reinforcer.

Note

- Prior to this task, the child should be able to complete each task individually.
- For visual learners, a pictured or written mini-plan of the individual tasks might be used.

- Placemats with outlines for a plate, a fork, a knife, and a spoon or chopsticks can be helpful for children completing chores.
- See an example picture activity schedule for chores in Figure 7.46.

Example Task 3: Recognizes Signal Words

- Child and therapist sit opposite each other.
- On the table is a stack of index cards with signal words written in capital letters, such as RESTROOM, MEN, WOMEN, ENTER, EXIT, PUSH, PULL.
- The therapist sets the timer for 20 seconds.
- The therapist presents the cards quickly, one at a time.
- Cards the child reads correctly are acknowledged and placed in one pile.
- Cards read incorrectly are put in another pile.
- The therapist and child practice the incorrect words prior to the next fluency check.
- The child counts the number of correct and incorrect cards and adds the data to a cumulative chart.
- After an improvement of his or her previous performance, the child receives a token.
- After the child receives three tokens, he or she receives a reinforcer.

Prerequisite
A prerequisite of the task is that the child understand and read the words on the cards individually.

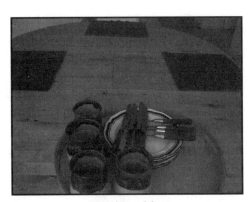

Set the table.

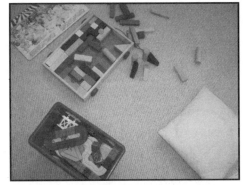

Put the toys away.

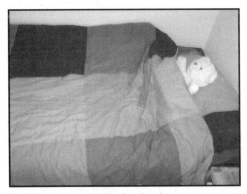

Make the bed.

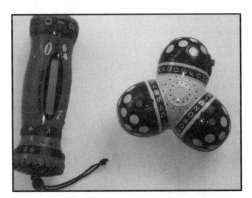

Finished! Now you can play.

FIGURE 7.46. Activity schedules help children with ASD better understand how to assist with household chores.

Notes

- The described see–say task (reading) should follow a hear–say task (language comprehension) and a see–do task.
- Photos of signal words found in the real environment can be used.
- Generalization of reading the signs in the real environment should be assessed.

Related Literature

Azrin, N., & Foxx, R. M. (1981). *Toilet training in less than a day.* New York: Pocket Books.

Baker, B. L., Brightman, A. J., Blacher, J. B., Heifez, L. J., Hinshaw, S. R., Murphy, D. M., et al. (2004). *Steps to independence: Teaching everyday skills to children with special needs* (4th ed.). Baltimore: Brookes.

Hodgdon, L. A. (2000). *Visual strategies for improving communication: Practical supports for school and home.* Troy, MI: QuirkRoberts.

McClannahan, L. E., & Krantz, P. J. (1999). *Activity schedules for children with autism: Teaching independent behavior.* Bethesda, MD: Woodbine House.

Von Gontard, A. (2004). *Enkopresis. Erscheinungsformen–Diagnostik–Therapie.* Stuttgart, Germany: Kohlhammer.

STEP Training Overview Forms

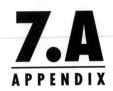

7.A

APPENDIX

STEP Training Overview:
Attention, Eye Contact, and Joint Attention

Child _____ Teacher _____

❐ Pretest   ❐ Posttest

Attention, Eye Contact, and Joint Attention Skill	Task	Date Tested	Child's Response +	Child's Response −	Notes
To give attention					
When called or addressed					
As request for					
Person					
Object					
Action					
Help					
As expression of					
Greeting					
Parting					
Surprise					
Joy					
Anxiety					
As question					
What is it?					
Where is it?					
Who has it?					
As spontaneous directed gaze					
To follow pointing					

Note. (+) = correct; (−) = incorrect.

© 2007 by PRO-ED, Inc.

**STEP Training Overview:
Matching and Sorting**

Child _____ Teacher _____

❐ Pretest   ❐ Posttest

Matching and Sorting Skill	Materials (circle those tested)	Date Tested	Child's Response		Other Materials Tested
			+	**−**	

Identical objects	Dishes and utensils
	  Cups, plates, bowls
	  Spoons, forks, knives
	Toys
	  Duplo or Lego blocks
	  Cars, ping-pong balls
	School and office supplies
	  Pencils, papers, cards
	  Paper clips
	Clothing
	  Shoes, socks
	Other:				

Objects that belong together	Dishes and utensils
	  Toothbrush and toothpaste
	  Pot and lid
	  Hammer and nail
	Toys
	  Toy car and garage
	  Train and tracks
	School and office supplies
	  Pencil and sharpener
	  Scissors and paper
	Clothing
	  Shoes and socks
	Other:				

Categories	Vehicles Food, drink Clothing Dolls, animals, furniture Office supplies Other:				
Puzzles (Two or more items per category)	Inset puzzle (with pictures of common objects) with 4 pieces Inset puzzle with 10 pieces Interlocking puzzle with pieces of varying complexity Other:				
Pictures to pictures (Identical)	Photos Cartoons or line drawings Lottery matching game cards Other:				

(continues)

© 2007 by PRO-ED, Inc.

Matching and Sorting Skill	Materials (circle those tested)	Date Tested	Child's Response		Other Materials Tested
			+	−	
Objects to pictures	Photos Cartoons or line drawings Other:				
Pictures to objects	Photos Cartoons or line drawings Other:				
Colors	Plastic chips, beads, color-boards, puzzles Worksheets Other:				
Shapes	Shape-sorters, beads Worksheets Other:				
Sizes and lengths	Size-boards, size-sorters, puzzles Shoes, plates, books Miniature objects Worksheets Other:				
Letters and words	Letter-boards Magnetic, plastic, wooden letters Stamps Word games, chips, cards Worksheets Other:				
Numbers	Number-boards Magnetic, plastic, wooden numbers Stamps Number games, chips, cards Worksheets Other:				
Amounts	Dominoes, number games Worksheets Other:				
Combinations	Color–shape Color–size Shape–size Shape–color Amounts Three or four combinations Other:				

(continues)

© 2007 by PRO-ED, Inc.

Matching and Sorting Skill	Materials (circle those tested)	Date Tested	Child's Response		Other Materials Tested
			+	−	
Persons	Illustrations Photos Cutouts Puzzles Lottery games Other:				
Emotions	Illustrations Photos Cutouts Other:				
Assembling objects	Flashlight Battery-operated toys Model cars Screws and nuts Pens Other:				
Storing objects	Toys School supplies Office supplies Groceries Other:				

Note. (+) = correct; (−) = incorrect.

© 2007 by PRO-ED, Inc.

**STEP Training Overview:
Imitation**

Child _____ Teacher _____

❏ Pretest ❏ Posttest

Imitation Skill	Task	Date Tested	Child's Response +	Child's Response −	Notes
Movements with an object	Place marble in bucket Use noisemaker Put on cap, sunglasses Move a toy car, animal, puppet				
Sequences of movement with two objects	First use a hammer, then move a car First comb hair, then blow nose First spray window, then spray a mirror				
A body movement	Clap hands Raise arms Nod				
Sequences of body movements	First touch head, then touch belly First crawl, then run				
Built and pictured models	Create blocks model Create Duplo and Lego model Present picture of house, table, people				
Lines, letters, numbers	Draw horizontal, vertical, diagonal lines Draw cross, circle, half-circle Write letters *L, T, F, E, A, M, N* Write letters *C, D, O, Q, G, P, R*				
Oral–motor, lip, tongue movements	Smack lips Smile Poke out tongue				
Facial expression, gestures, body positions	Make happy, sad face Gesture for "Come here," "Quiet"				
Sounds, syllables, words, speech melody	Say, "Hua-hua" (Native American chant) Make dog and cat sounds Make "aaa," "ooo," "uuu," "eee" sounds Make "m," "b," "p," "d," "t" sounds Say, "Mama," "Dada," "up," "go"				
Sentences, songs, scripts	Say, "Want ball, candy" Sing language songs Say, "Ready, steady, go!"				

Note. (+) = correct; (−) = incorrect.

© 2007 by PRO-ED, Inc.

STEP Training Overview:
Language Comprehension

Child _____ Teacher _____

❐ Pretest   ❐ Posttest

Language Comprehension Skill	Task Examples	Date Tested	Child's Response		Notes
			+	−	
One-step instructions with objects	"Put in." "Ready, set, go." "One, two, and the last number is ... three!" "Eat the cookie." "Drink the juice."				
One-step instructions without objects	"Come here." "Sit down." "Stand up." "Wait." "Line up."				
Objects	"Where is the ball?" "Get the teddy bear."				
People	"Pass the spoon to Mommy." "The cookie is with Dad."				
Actions and object functions	"Throw the ball." "Run." "Make the bear bounce." "Which one can you eat with?" "Get something to build."				
Body parts	"Put lotion on your face." "Pat your tummy."				
Related multiple-step instructions	"Put the milk in the fridge." "Get the scissors and cut."				
Unrelated multiple-step instructions	"Put the animals on the truck." "Put the chairs on the table and turn on the light."				
Categories	"Take a vehicle." "Take a piece of fruit."				
Sounds	"What did you hear?" (sort pictures to taped sounds)				
Locations	"The chips are in the living room." "Go to the playground."				
Adjectives Color Size Shape Number Amount Opposites	"Take a pink Smartie." "The car is in the big box." "Which sign is square?" "Take two cookies." "Take the full (or empty) glass." "Carry the heavy (or light) bag."				

(continues)

© 2007 by PRO-ED, Inc.

Language Comprehension Skill	Task Examples	Date Tested	Child's Response		Notes
			+	**−**	
Emotions	"Which child is happy?" "Show an angry face."				
Gender	"Line up with the boys."				
Singular and plural	"Eat one candy." "Eat many candies." "Where is your foot?" "Where are your feet?"				
Prepositions	"Sit in (or on or next to) the box."				
Pronouns	"Brush my (or your) hair." "Shake his (or her) hand."				

Questions
  What?
  Who?
  Where?
  How?
  Which?
  Why?
	"What is the boy eating?" "Who is wearing a hat?" "Where is the rabbit?" "How does the ice cream taste?" "Which bag belongs to you?" "Why is the boy crying?"				

Notes

- The above tasks are listed according to developmental sequence and level of difficulty.

- The actual task sequence followed should match the needs, interests, and settings of the child.

- Training steps can be changed and additional tasks can be added.

- Language comprehension and language expression can be trained at the same time.

- The tasks can be done with real people, objects, and events in addition to dolls, animals, miniature objects, pictures, and picture symbols.

Note. (+) = correct; (−) = incorrect.

© 2007 by PRO-ED, Inc.

STEP Training Overview:
Active Communication

Child _____ Teacher _____

☐ Pretest   ☐ Posttest

Communication Function	Task	Date Tested	Child's Response		Notes
			+	**−**	
Request	Therapist: "What do you want?" "Who do you want?" "Which one do you want? Child: "I want _____."				
Objects					
Food and drink	Chips, cookie, M&M, banana, rice, juice, milk				
Toys	Bubbles, ball, balloon, yo-yo, sand, water, television, computer				
Clothing	Shoes, socks, jacket, pants				
People and names	Mom, Dad, sister, brother, grandparents				
Actions	Eat, drink, play, swing, come, go, color, in and out (with puzzle), on and off (with battery-operated toys)				
Object features	Red, blue, big, small _____				
Expression	Therapist: "Do you want this?"				
Affirmation	Child: "Yes," "Sure," "Okay"				
Rejection	Child: "No," "Don't want"				
Denial	Child: "No"				
Description and labeling	Therapist: "What is this?" "This is _____?"				
Objects	Child:				
Food	Apple, orange, cake, vegetable, meat, fish				
Toys	Car, bus, train, Lego, block, doll, Teddy, music, bike				
Household items	Bed, chair, table, toilet, TV				
Utensils	Spoon, cup, crayon				
Clothing	Shoes, socks, pants, shirt				
Vehicles	Car, bus, scooter, bike				
Locations	Bedroom, bathroom, playground, kindergarten, school				

(*continues*)

© 2007 by PRO-ED, Inc.

Communication Function	Task	Date Tested	Child's Response		Notes
			+	**−**	
People Names	Therapist: "Who is it?" Child: Names of mother, father, sister, brother, therapist				
Body parts	Therapist: "What is it?" Child: "Hair," "Teeth," "Nose," "Mouth," "Eyes," "Hand," "Feet"				
Emotions	Therapist: "How does he (or she) feel?" Child: "Happy," "Sad," "Angry," "Scared"				
Actions and object functions	Therapist: "What am I doing?" "(Object) is for (action)." Child: "Eating," "Drinking," "Opening," "Closing," "Putting on," "Taking off," "Combing," "Washing," "Coloring," "Cutting," "Riding"				
Animals	Therapist: "What is this?" "What makes this sound?" Child: "Dog," "Cat," "Bird," "Horse," "Cow," "Elephant"				
Greetings and farewells	Child: "Hi," "Hello," "Bye"				
Object features	Therapist: "Tell me about the _____." "This is a _____." "What color is the _____?" "What size are the _____?" Child:				
Color Size Opposites	"Red," "Blue" "Big," "Little" "Hot," "Cold," "One," "Many"				
Questions	Interesting objects are hidden and the child is prompted to ask for them. Therapist: "Ask about the cookie (or bag or flashlight)." Child:				
"What" "Who" "Where"	"What is it?" "What's inside?" "Who has it?" "Where is it?"				
Use social scripts	Objects are withheld until the child uses pleasantries or requests help to get access to liked items. Child: "Please," "Thank you," "Thanks," "Help"				

Note. (+) = correct; (−) = incorrect.

© 2007 by PRO-ED, Inc.

**STEP Training Overview:
Expanded Communication**

Child _____   Teacher _____

❏ Pretest ❏ Posttest

Expanded Communication and Vocabulary Skills	Task Examples	Date Tested	Child's Response +	Child's Response −	Notes
Spontaneity					
Objects					
Food					
Toys					
Household items					
School					
Traffic					
Utensils					
People					
Relatives					
Professions					
Body parts					
Feelings					
Living things					
Pets					
Farm animals					
Zoo animals					
Sea animals					
Birds					
Plants					
Trees					
Actions					
Food and drinks					
Toys and games					
Household					
School					
Traffic					
Utensils					
Functions					
Objects					
Body parts					
Locations					

(continues)

© 2007 by PRO-ED, Inc.

Expanded Communication and Vocabulary Skills	Task Examples	Date Tested	Child's Response		Notes
			+	−	
Belonging					
Objects					
Locations					
Categories					
More-word utterances					
Plurals					
Comparatives					
Knowledge					
Food and drinks					
Vehicles					
Professions					
Animals					
Calendar and time					
Time (adverbs such as *today, yesterday, tomorrow, soon, finally*)					
Prepositions					
Pronouns					
Personal					
Possessive					
Demonstrative					
Questions					
When?					
How?					
Who?					
Which?					
Why?					
Language functions					
Greetings, farewells					
Instructions, orders					
Comments					
Interjections					
Corrections					

(*continues*)

© 2007 by PRO-ED, Inc.

Expanded Communication and Vocabulary Skills	Task Examples	Date Tested	Child's Response		Notes
			+	−	
Reciprocal communication					
Past, present, future					
Social scripts and compliments					
Conversation					
Name					
Age					
Address					
School					
Family					
Hobbies					
Sports					
Television, computer					

Note. (+) = correct; (−) = incorrect.

© 2007 by PRO-ED, Inc.

STEP Training Overview:
Play and Social Behavior

Child _____ Teacher _____

❏ Pretest ❏ Posttest

Play and Social Behavior Skills	Task Examples	Date Tested	Child's Response +	Child's Response –	Notes
Appropriate isolated play	Plays appropriately with:				
Sensory play	• Bubbles, tops, sand, and water toys				
Cause–effect play	• Jack-in-the-box, wind-up toys, busy boxes				
Construction play	• Duplo or Lego bricks, marble run, play-dough				
Imaginary play	• Vehicles, animals, people figures, dolls				
Parallel play	Plays parallel to another child for at least 10 minutes				
Eye contact and joint attention	Looks to where other children look (e.g., when the teacher reads a storybook, when other children wait in line for equipment at the playground)				
Cooperative play					
• Turn taking	Throws the balloon, ball, or Frisbee back and forth to another child; pushes car or bus back and forth to another child; takes turn building a tower; waits for his or her turn during basketball				
• Sharing	Shares toys such as cars, crayons, or zoo animals				
• Offering toys	Offers missing puzzle piece; offers cutter for cutting play-dough				
• Giving in	Indicates verbally or nonverbally that someone else can have a turn, take the toy, or be the leader				
• Losing	The following sentiments are indicated verbally or nonverbally: "It's okay to lose or be second." "Too bad, I can win next time"				
Imitates others	Imitates others during songs or shadow or mirror games; while constructing with blocks; during cutting, pasting, and play-dough activities; or when joining a game on the playground				

© 2007 by PRO-ED, Inc.

(continues)

Play and Social Behavior Skills	Task Examples	Date Tested	Child's Response		Notes
			+	**−**	
Shows interest in other children • Comments • Questions	Comments or asks questions when observing or when involved in games with peers, such as the following: • "You are drawing (or building) an airplane!" • "Can I try (or have or borrow) this?" • "What do you think about my picture (or essay)?" • "Is this right (or good)?"				
Reacts to instructions of other children and instructs others • Follows instruction • Repeats instructions • Instructs • Takes on tasks and roles	 Simon says: "Everybody hops on one leg …" Repeats instruction until the other child responds Assigns tasks and roles to other children, such as the following: • "You clean up the books (or animals)." • "You are the policeman (or teacher or student)." • "I'm the fireman (or driver)." • "I'll get the tracks (or cars or crayons)."				
Considers others' perspectives • Wishes • Interests and hobbies • Fears • Prerequisite knowledge	 Serves others according to their likes and wishes in the role-play games of "restaurant" or "toy store" Asks others in a "reporter" game about their interests and hobbies Asks others about their wishes and fears Introduces topics and gives missing information				
Considers rules • Rule-governed games • Explicit social rules	 Complies with rules in board, sports, or party games Recognizes in cartoons and role-play how to behave appropriately during the following situations: • Greetings and good-byes				

(continues)

© 2007 by PRO-ED, Inc.

Play and Social Behavior Skills	Task Examples	Date Tested	Child's Response +	Child's Response −	Notes
Considers rules (*cont.*)					
• Explicit social rules (*cont.*)	• Saying "thanks (or thank you or you're welcome or excuse me)"				
	• Waiting instead of interrupting				
• Hidden rules	• Not talking about topics about which the other person is not interested				
	• Not being overly blunt				
	• Adapting behavior and word choice to the setting or the interaction partner (e.g., behaving in a different way at home; at school; in the doctor's office; on the telephone; and toward parents, teachers, peers, friends, and strangers)				
Understands and expresses feelings					
• Facial expression and gesture	Sorts, matches, recognizes, and labels pictures with emotional expressions such as disappointed, frustrated, afraid, terrified, nervous, excited				
	Labels emotions in pictures, role-play, puppet play, and stories				
• Cause and effect	Knows what people feel when they get praised, scolded, or mobbed, or when they lose something or somebody				
	Knows why someone gets praised, scolded, loved, liked, disliked				
	Gives reasons for emotions such as disappointment, frustration, fear, nervousness, excitement				
Develops perspectives and empathy					
• Role-play	Participates in role-play, taking on different roles				
• Identification	Pretends that toy animals, people, dolls have lives of their own				
• Empathy	Shows joy when someone pretends to get a present				
	Shows sympathy when someone pretends to cry or be hurt				

(continues)

© 2007 by PRO-ED, Inc.

Play and Social Behavior Skills	Task Examples	Date Tested	Child's Response +	Child's Response −	Notes
Offers and gives help	Offers help when someone carries too much or seems hurt Does chores such as setting the table				
Gives and receives compliments	Gives compliment, expresses gratitude, or gives additional information such as the following: • "I really like your eraser." • "Thanks!" • "Oh yes, I just got these shoes yesterday."				
Initiates play and social interaction	Indicates interest in others, joins others, initiates contact such as the following: • "Hi, my name is _____." "What's your name?" • "Do you also play _____?" • "Do you want to come to _____?" • "Can I join?"				
Takes and gives feedback and criticism	• "Sorry, I didn't mean to _____." "Excuse me." • "Okay, I can fix this." • "This is too difficult (or easy or noisy)." • "This makes me nervous."				
Solves problems	Recognizes the problem (e.g., noise during P.E.) and selects a solution from various alternatives • "I need a break (or a drink or my headphone)." • "I can wait." • "I'd better call to say I'm late."				

Note. (+) = correct; (−) = incorrect.

© 2007 by PRO-ED, Inc.

STEP Training Overview:
Self-Help Skills and Independence

Child _____ Teacher _____

❒ Pretest ❒ Posttest

Self-Help Skills	Task Examples	Date Tested	Child's Response +	Child's Response −	Notes
Meals and snacks					
• Eating	• Eats small pieces of food by hand • Eats a snack or meal by hand • Eats with spoon • Eats with knife and fork				
• Drinking	• Drinks from a training cup • Drinks from a regular cup				
• Sandwich making	• Spreads butter on bread • Adds meat, cheese • Cuts bread in half				
• Drink preparation	• Prepares simple drink (e.g., lemonade, chocolate milk)				
• Simple meal preparation	• Prepares cereal, toast				
Toileting					
• Dryness	• Stays dry and clean during the day when regularly sent to the toilet • Stays dry and clean during the day, but has occasional accidents at night • Does not have accidents during the day or at night				
• Wiping	• Wipes herself or himself				
• Flushing	• Flushes the toilet				
• Clothing refastening	• Refastens clothing after toileting (e.g., buttons, zipper)				
Personal hygiene					
• Hands	• Washes and dries hands				
• Face	• Washes and dries face				
• Teeth	• Brushes teeth				
• Hair	• Combs hair • Washes and dries hair				
• Shower and bath	• Takes a shower or bath and dries off				

(continues)

© 2007 by PRO-ED, Inc.

Self-Help Skills	Task Examples	Date Tested	Child's Response +	Child's Response −	Notes
Dressing and undressing					
• Socks, shoes	• Takes off shoes, socks • Puts on shoes, socks • Unties, ties shoes				
• Shorts, pants	• Takes off shorts, pants • Puts on shorts, pants				
• T-shirt, sweater	• Takes off t-shirt, sweater • Puts on t-shirt, sweater				
• Buttons	• Unfastens big, small buttons • Fastens big, small buttons				
• Zipper	• Opens zipper of pants or skirt • Closes zipper of pants or skirt • Opens zipper of jacket				
Household chores					
• Table setting	• Sets table for _____ persons with dishes and utensils				
• Laundry	• Puts laundry into washing machine				
• Bed making	• Makes own bed				
• Bathroom cleaning	• Cleans shower, bathtub				
Independence					
• Shopping	• Buys one or several items by himself or herself				
• Signal words	• Recognizes signal words such as *Restroom, Men, Women, Enter, Exit, Stop, Push, Pull*				
• Telephone	• Answers the phone appropriately • Calls familiar and unfamiliar people				
• Money	• Gives money to cashier • Expects change • Buys snack or drink from machine				
• Orientation	• Knows rooms of own home • Finds liked item in the house • Moves around neighborhood, childcare center, school • Finds liked item in a familiar supermarket • Finds parents' car in —familiar parking lot —unfamiliar parking lot				

(*continues*)

© 2007 by PRO-ED, Inc.

Self-Help Skills	Task Examples	Date Tested	Child's Response		Notes
			+	−	
Independence (*cont.*)					
• Traffic	• Walks or drives on correct side of street				
	• Responds to traffic lights				
	• Crosses street appropriately				
	• Behaves appropriately in school or on public bus				
• Time	• Recognizes time, including hour, half hour, quarter hour, and minutes				
	• Tells time, hour, half hour, quarter hour, and minutes				
	• Tells time on digital and analog clocks				
	• Knows what happens at what time at home and in school				
	• Knows days of the week				
	• Knows what happens in what month or season				

Note. (+) = correct; (−) = incorrect.

© 2007 by PRO-ED, Inc.

Blank Data Forms for the Four Teaching Methods

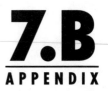

APPENDIX

Data Form for Discrete Trial Format

Child _____

Skill Area _____   Teacher _____

In addition to recording the child's performance, indicate specifics about the task setup, such as the number of distractors, types of prompts, and reinforcer schedule. Try to conduct about 10 trials per date and five sessions per week. Note that if the child fails to respond, the response should be scored as incorrect. Plot data on daily learning graphs.

Target Skill	Task Setup		Prompt	Consequence	Date	Trials (+) or (−)											% Correct
	Material or Task	Instruction															

© 2007 by PRO-ED, Inc.

Data Form for Precision Teaching

Child _____

Teacher _____

Skill Area _____

| Target Skill | Task Setup | | Time Unit | Consequence | Level of Task Hierarchy | Date | Observations
Number of correct and incorrect responses per time unit | Fluency Aim |
	Material or Task	Instruction						

Note. Level of Task Hierarchy should be filled in with the type of task: See–do, Hear–do, Hear–say, or See–say.

© 2007 by PRO-ED, Inc.

Data Form for Natural and Experience-Based Teaching

Child _____

Teacher _____

Skill Area _____

Target Skill	Task Setup		Date	Observations (p, e, or f)					% Passed
	Material or Task	Instruction		1	2	3	4	5	

Note. p = passing; e = emerging; f = failing.

© 2007 by PRO-ED, Inc.

Data Form for Visual Learning

Child _____   Teacher _____

Skill Area _____

Target Skill	Task	Instruction		Consequence	Date	Child's Response		
		Verbal	Visual			p	e	f

Note. **p** = passing; **e** = emerging; **f** = failing.

© 2007 by PRO-ED, Inc.

Setting Up a Home Therapy Program

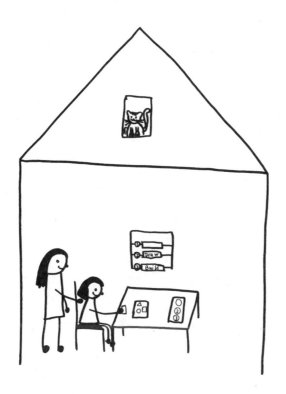

Chapter Overview

Importance of a Home Program

Who Can Train Children with ASD?

Organization of the Home Program

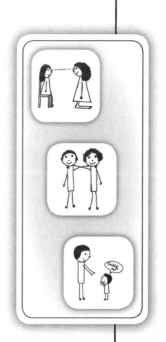

E ver since the early studies by Ivar Lovaas (1987), intensive behavioral training programs have been considered a crucial component of early intervention in young children with ASD (see the recommendations of the New York State Department, 1999; Perry & Condillac, 2003). Trained therapists will usually conduct these behavioral training programs in the child's home for 18 to 40 hours per week for at least 2 years. Because of the success of early home-based intervention, various private companies now offer these programs in many regions.

Parents' reactions to home-based intervention are mixed. Some parents enjoy having the support of young and dynamic therapists in their home environment, while others consider this an invasion of privacy and an additional source of stress. There are parents who would like professional in-home support, but do not have access to experienced supervisors and a team of proficient therapists; others feel overwhelmed by the effort involved in organizing such a program, securing funding, or paying for it outright.

IMPORTANCE OF A HOME PROGRAM

For parents struggling with the decision of whether to get involved in a home therapy program with their child, the following information may be helpful: The duration of the program, the specific methods used, and the training of the parents themselves play a crucial role in the child's progress. In one of the studies replicating the early intervention research conducted by Lovaas, 24 children between the ages of 25 and 42 months were divided into three different groups. One group received parent-directed treatment, one received intensive clinic intervention, and another received nonspecific treatment. Results after 1 year showed the following: Even though the parents in the first group received only 6 hours of supervision per month and conducted an irregular number of therapy hours per week, the children's IQs increased an average of 18 points. Children in the second group, who participated in a 40-hours-per-week clinic training, showed an average increase of 23 IQ points, which is only slightly better than the children in the parent group. The third group of children, who were integrated into general education kindergarten classes and had an additional 4 to 6 hours of speech therapy or occupational therapy each week, showed an average decrease of 8 IQ points (Sallows & Graupner, 1999).

Children in the parent-directed training group and the clinic group also showed significant improvement in their language. Prior to the training, 46% of the whole cohort was nonverbal, 46% used only a few words, and 8% ($n = 2$) talked in three-word or more sentences. After a year of training, the figures for the nonverbal group of children looked very different. The percentage of nonverbal children had dropped to 17%. Of the original nonverbal group, 12% now used single words and 71% had developed three-word and more utterances. Even though this research leaves some questions unanswered, such as the comparability of the three groups and the exact number of hours parents spent in therapeutic interactions with their children, it does show that parent training and behavior intervention are important components in a child's progress.

The benefits of home-based intervention programs involving parents were also evident in another study involving eight children with ASD, ages 28 to 44 months (Bernard-Opitz et al., 2004). At the National University of Singapore, the Behavioral Intervention Center for Children provided a program where parents were trained to work with their children for 10 hours per week. A team of 10 psychology students, who were trained in behavioral methods, supported the parents. The university students also worked with each child at home for another 10 hours per week. To ensure that behavioral methods were implemented and teaching targets were functional, trained research assistants and the author supervised the students in vivo as well as through analysis of video recordings of training sessions. Based on pre- and postvideo assessment, it was established that six of the eight children improved significantly in compliance, attention, communication, and play. Progress was less obvious for two of the children who had a developmental age below 12 months and whose parents were the least involved of the group. For five of the eight children, scores on the *Symbolic Play Test* (Lowe & Costello, 1988) increased by 8.1 months over the observation period. Scores on the *Prelinguistic Autism Diagnostic Schedule* (DiLavore et al., 1995), the standard observation test for autistic children, also reflected a surprising improvement. After 10 weeks of therapy, seven of the eight children showed reduced autism scores (Bernard-Opitz et al., 2004).

In addition to the above-mentioned benefits, there are several practical reasons why a home program is important for children with ASD. To make sure that therapy goals for each child are relevant and that methods are matched to the daily environment, therapists must involve parents, siblings, and—in some cases—extended family and family friends. Not only does this ensure that teaching targets are related to the child's daily experiences, but it also ensures that they are generalized to her or his home environment (L. Koegel, Koegel, & Dunlap, 1996). Young children especially spend a large amount of their time at home and often have highly motivated family members. This motivation can be effectively translated into positive strides for the child if work is carried out at home. Moreover, because parents usually control the most powerful reinforcers, they are undoubtedly significant in the child's behavior management regime.

WHO CAN TRAIN CHILDREN WITH ASD?

Not everyone makes a good therapist, and not all parents are excited about training their own children. An increasing number of parents work full-time and cannot afford to give up that work to be involved with their child for an extensive number of hours. These parents may opt for private home tutors or recognized behavioral companies to support home-based intervention. For both options, the therapists should have a background in behavioral intervention methods and psychology as well as supervised experience with autistic children.

On the other hand, many parents are capable of combining a high degree of sensitivity for their children with excellent therapeutic skills and knowledge. These parents can be very successful therapists for their own children. The involvement of siblings, other relatives, neighbors, students, and friends should be encouraged, and, as described in the integrated playgroups discussion in Chapter 7, siblings and peers can be highly effective models. Other volunteers can oversee behavioral programs or provide assistance with data taking or video recording. In all cases, it is important to coordinate behavior management and intervention strategies, organize material and learning data, and seek qualified supervision.

ORGANIZATION OF THE HOME PROGRAM

Parents who want to set up their own intensive home program should participate in structured parent training. They should seek supervision by experienced therapists with a behavioral background who specialize in autism. By advertising at neighboring universities, contacting lecturers in psychology, psychiatry, or education, and garnering the support of relatives, friends, and community members, parents should be able to attain a pool of 5 to 10 therapists. Figure 8.1 shows a sample advertisement. It may be more cost-effective for some parents to involve university students who are carrying out their clinical placement or participating in applied research studies. Once a supervisor knowledgeable in the basics of behavior analysis and intervention has trained the team, specific structured and experience-based teaching methods must be taught to the parents and other team members using role-play, possibly with video feedback. For the development of therapy goals, the child's Individualized Education Program can serve as a guideline. In addition, the STEP curriculum presented here and the listed references can

---

Home Therapist Needed

Needed: Students to work under professional supervision, at least 2 hours per week, with my 4-year-old autistic child.

What can you get out of this?
- The feeling of having contributed to significant changes in a child's life
- An introduction to behavior therapy and autism
- Weekly team supervision
- Practicum hours

Where?
- At our home, 24 Rose Lane

When and for how long?
- Immediately
- For at least 8 weeks

I look forward to your call.

Tania Miller
555-7346

FIGURE 8.1. A sample advertisement for hiring a home therapy team.

be helpful. Therapy targets should be agreed upon with the parents, the school, and all home therapists involved. Some parents have excellent organizational skills that can support activities such as finding team members and organizing team meetings and daily data. Team meetings with the supervisor should be conducted at least once a week.

A home-based intervention program can vary in intensity. Families should decide on the number of therapy hours per day, the frequency of supervision and team meetings, and the number of therapists.

A home therapy program can consist of any or all of the four STEP methods: discrete trial training, precision teaching, natural and experience-based learning, and visual learning. While one family may prefer experience-based or play-oriented methods, another may enjoy a structured daily program with planned activities for developing concepts, communication, play, social and self-help behavior, and even leisure activities.

Whatever the situation, all decisions should be made with a view to the long-term improvement of the lives of the child and her or his family. Parents are the people to whom the child is most closely related and should therefore be respected as specialists of that child. We, as professionals, are members of a team that can contribute knowledge about autism and its treatment, but do not have to live with the results of interventions in the same way as the families do.

Conclusion

I hope that this book, and the STEP curriculum described within its pages, will help parents, therapists, and teachers who live and work with children with ASD. My desire is that because of this manual, it will become common practice for intervention programs to be matched to the unique needs and interests of the individual child. Instead of waiting for miracles to happen, all parties involved should collaborate to find an effective teaching program that will allow the child to be successful. This book aims to contribute to this process by providing a spectrum of evidence-based teaching methods and a curriculum full of functional and motivating steps. Specific strategies have been demonstrated that will help the reader to provide a tailor-made program, taking into consideration the child's skill, learning, and behavior profile—a process that will benefit all children with ASD. My ultimate hope is that some children not only will reach the expected developmental stages, but will progress rapidly. You may witness an amazing spurt of development or simply one small precious step at a time—changes in your child that may well border on the miraculous.

References

Abrams, P., & Henriques, L. (2004). *The autistic spectrum parents' daily helper: A workbook for you and your child.* Berkeley, CA: Ulysses Press.

American Psychiatric Association. (1994). *Diagnostic and statistical manual of mental disorders* (4th ed.). Washington, DC: Author.

American Psychological Association. (2002). Criteria for evaluating treatment guidelines. *American Psychologist, 57,* 1052–1059.

Asperger, H. (1944). Die 'autistischen psychopathen' im kindesalter. *Archiv für Psychiatrie und Nervenkrankheiten, 117,* 76–136.

Ayres, J. (1979). *Sensory integration and the child.* Los Angeles: Western Psychological Services.

Azrin, N., & Foxx, R. M. (1981). *Toilet training in less than a day.* New York: Pocket Books.

Baer, D. M., Wolf, M. M., & Risley, T. R. (1968). Some current dimensions of applied behaviour analysis. *Journal of Applied Behavior Analysis, 1,* 91–97.

Baker, B. L., Brightman, A. J., Blacher, J. B., Heifez, L. J., Hinshaw, S. R., Murphy, D. M., et al. (2004). *Steps to independence: Teaching everyday skills to children with special needs* (4th ed.). Baltimore: Brookes.

Baranek, G. T. (2002). Efficacy of sensory and motor interventions for children with autism. *Journal of Autism and Developmental Disorders, 32,* 397–422.

Barkley, R. A. (2006). *Attention-deficit hyperactivity disorder: A handbook for diagnosis and treatment* (3rd ed.). New York: Guilford.

Baron-Cohen, S., Allen, J., & Gillberg, C. (1992). Can autism be detected at 18 months? The needle, the haystack, and the CHAT. *British Journal of Psychiatry, 166,* 839–843.

Baron-Cohen, S., Leslie, A. M., & Frith, U. (1985). Does the autistic child have a "Theory of Mind"? *Cognition, 21,* 37–46.

Bayley, N. (1993). *Bayley Scales of Infant Development* (2nd ed.). San Antonio, TX: Psychological Corp.

Berard, G. (1993). *Hearing equals behavior* (Trans.). New Canaan, CT: Keats.

Berk, L. E. (1989). *Child development.* Needham Heights, MA: Allyn & Bacon.

Bernard-Opitz, V. (1981). *Developmental and behavioral approaches in training children with autism.* Unpublished doctoral dissertation, University of Göttingen, Germany.

Bernard-Opitz V. (1983, August). *Communicative effectiveness in nonverbal autistic and mentally retarded children.* Paper presented at the annual conference of the American Psychological Association, Anaheim, CA.

Bernard-Opitz, V. (1985, August). *Counter-control problems of autistic children: Analysis and cognitive intervention.* Poster session presented at the annual conference of the American Psychological Association, Los Angeles, CA.

Bernard-Opitz, V. (1993, June). The STEP program. *Autism News Singapore,* 9–10.

Bernard-Opitz, V. (2005). Precision teaching: Making learning effortless. *Autism News of Orange County and the Rest of the World,* 9–10.

Bernard-Opitz, V., Blesch, G., & Holz, K. (1988). *Sprachlos muß keiner bleiben: Handzeichen und andere Kommunikationshilfen für autistisch und geistig Behinderte.* Freiburg im Breisgau, Freiburg, Germany: Lambertus Verlag.

Bernard-Opitz, V., Blesch, G., & Holz, K. (1992). *Sprachlos muß keiner bleiben: Handzeichen und andere Kommunikationshilfen für autistisch und geistig Behinderte.* Freiburg im Breisgau (2nd ed.), Freiburg, Germany: Lambertus Verlag.

Bernard-Opitz, V., Ing, S., & Tan, Y. K. (2004). Comparison of behavioral and natural play interventions for young children with autism. *Autism: The International Journal of Research and Practice, 8*(3), 319–334.

Bernard-Opitz, V., Sriram, N., & Sapuan, S. (1999). Enhancing vocal imitations in children with autism using the IBM SpeechViewer. *Autism: The International Journal of Research and Practice, 3*(2), 131–149.

Bettison, S. (1996). The long-term effects of auditory training on children with autism. *Journal of Autism and Developmental Disorders, 26,* 361–374.

Beyer, J., & Gammeltoft, L. (2003). *Autism and play.* London: Kingsley.

Biklen, D. (1993). *Communication unbound.* New York: Teachers College Press.

Binder, C., & Watkins, C. L. (1990). Precision teaching and direct instruction: Measurably superior instructional technology in schools. *Performance Improvement Quarterly, 3*(4), 74–96.

Blank, M., McKirdy, L. S., & Payne, P. (2000). *Links to language.* Upper Montclair, NJ: HELP Associates.

Bloom, P. (2000). *How children learn the meanings of words.* Cambridge, MA: MIT Press.

Bölte, S., & Poustka, F. (2002a). The relation between general cognitive level and adaptive behavior domains in individuals with autism with and without co-morbid mental retardation. *Child Psychiatry and Human Development, 33*(2), 165–172.

Bölte, S., & Poustka, F. (2002b). Intervention bei autistischen Störungen: Status quo, evidenzbasierte, fragliche und fragwürdige Techniken. *Zeitschrift für Kinder- und Jugendpsychiatrie, 30*(4), 271–280.

Bondy, A., Dickey, D., & Buswell, S. (2002). *The pyramid approach to education: Lesson plans for young children.* Newark, DE: Pyramid Educational Products.

Bondy, A., & Frost, L. (1994). The Picture Exchange Communication System. *Focus on Autistic Behavior, 9,* 1–19.

Boswell, S. (2006). *Preschool curriculum guide.* Chapel Hill, NC: Division TEACCH, University of North Carolina.

Boswell, S., Reynolds, B., Faulkner, R., & Benson, M. (2006). *Let's get started! Visually structured tasks from the TEACCH Early Childhood Demonstration Program.* Chapel Hill, NC: Division TEACCH, University of North Carolina.

Braun, O. (2002). *Sprachstörungen bei Kindern und Jugendlichen: Diagnose, Therapie, Förderung.* Stuttgart, Germany: Kohlhammer.

Bricker, D., & Waddell, M. (2002). *AEPS curriculum for birth to three years.* Baltimore: Brookes.

Brigance, A. (2004). *Inventory of Early Development II.* North Billerica, MA: Curriculum Associates.

Brown, J. R., & Rogers, S. J. (2003). Cultural issues in autism. In S. Ozonoff, S. J. Rogers, & R. L. Hendren (Eds.), *Autism spectrum disorders: A research review for practitioners* (pp. 209–226). Washington, DC: American Psychiatric.

Brown, R. (1979). *A first language.* Cambridge, MA: Harvard University Press.

California Department of Developmental Services. (2000). *Changes in the population of persons with autism and pervasive developmental disorders in California's developmental services system: 1987 through 1998.* Retrieved October 9, 2006, from http://www.dds.cahwnet.gov/autism/pdf/autism_report_1999.pdf

Camarata, S. M. (2001). On the importance of integrating naturalistic language, social intervention, and speech-intelligibility training. In L. K. Koegel, R. L. Koegel, & G. Dunlap (Eds.), *Positive behavioral support* (pp. 333–351). Baltimore: Brookes.

Camp, B. W., & Bash, M. A. (1981). *Think aloud: Increasing social and cognitive skills—A problem-solving program for children.* Champaign, IL: Research Press.

Carr, E. G. (1982). Sign language. In R. L. Koegel, A. Rincover, & A. L. Egel (Eds.), *Educating and understanding autistic children* (pp. 142–157). San Diego, CA: College Hill Press.

Carr, E. G., Binkoff, J. A., Kologinsky, E., & Eddy, M. (1978). Acquisition of sign language by autistic children: Expressive labeling. *Journal of Applied Behavior Analysis, 11*(4), 489–501.

Carr, E. G., & Darcy, M. (1990). Setting generality of peer modeling in children with autism. *Journal of Autism and Developmental Disorders, 20*(1), 45–59.

Charlop-Christy, M. H., Carpenter, M., Le, L., LeBlanc, L. A., & Kellet, K. (2002). Using the Picture Exchange Communication System (PECS) with children with autism: Assessment of PECS acquisition, speech, social–communicative behavior, and problem behavior. *Journal of Applied Behavior Analysis, 35,* 213–231.

Chin, A., & Bernard-Opitz, V. (2000). Teaching conversational skills to children with autism: Effect on the development of a theory of mind. *Journal of Autism and Developmental Disorders, 30*(6), 569–583.

Clannahan, L. E., & Krantz, P. J. (1999). *Activity schedules for children with autism: Teaching independent behavior.* Bethesda, MD: Woodbine House.

Committee on Educational Interventions for Children with Autism, Division of Behavioral and Social Sciences and Education, National Research Council. (2001). *Educating children with autism.* Washington, DC: National Academy Press.

Dawson, G. (1989). *Autism: Nature, diagnosis and treatment.* New York: Guilford Press.

Dawson, G., & Osterling, J. (1997). Early intervention in autism. In M. J. Guralnick (Ed.), *The effectiveness of early intervention* (pp. 307–326). Baltimore: Brookes.

Dawson, G., & Watling, R. (2000). Interventions to facilitate auditory, visual, and motor integration in autism: A review of the evidence. *Journal of Autism and Developmental Disorders, 30*(5), 423–425.

Delprato, D. J. (2001). Comparisons of discrete-trial and normalized behavioral language intervention for young children with autism. *Journal of Autism and Developmental Disorders, 31*(3), 315–325.

DiLavore, P. C., Lord, C., & Rutter, M. (1995). The Pre-linguistic Autism Diagnostic Observation Schedule. *Journal of Autism and Developmental Disorders, 25*(4), 355–379.

Dilling, H., & Freyberger, H. J. (1999). *Taschenführer zur ICD-10 Klassifikation psychischer Störungen.* Bern, Germany: Verlag Hans Huber.

Dunlap, G., & Koegel, R. L. (1980). Motivating autistic children through stimulus variation. *Journal of Applied Behavior Analysis, 13*(4), 619–627.

Durand, M. (1998). *Sleep better! A guide to improving sleep for children with special needs.* Baltimore: Brookes.

Durand, M. V. (2004). Learned optimism. *Autism News of Orange County and the Rest of the World, 1*(2), 22.

Durand, V. M., & Crimmins, D. B. (1988). Identifying the variables maintaining self-injurious behavior. *Journal of Autism and Developmental Disorders, 18*(1), 99–117.

Durand, V. M., & Merges, E. (2001). Functional communication training: A contemporary behavior analytic intervention for problem behaviors. *Focus on Autism and Other Developmental Disabilities, 16,* 110–119.

Eckenrode, L., Fennell, P., & Hearsay, K. (2003). *Tasks galore: Creative ideas for teachers, therapists and parents working with exceptional children.* Raleigh, NC: Tasks Galore.

Eckenrode, L., Fennell, P., & Hearsay, K. (2004). *Tasks galore: For the real world.* Raleigh, NC: Tasks Galore.

Erles-Vollrath, T. L., Cook, K. T., & Ganz, J. B. (2006). *How to develop and implement visual supports.* Austin, TX: PRO-ED.

Fabrizio, M. A., & Ferris, K. J. (2003, May). *Overview of fluency-based instruction for learners with autism.* Workshop at the annual convention of the CalABA, San Francisco, CA.

Fabrizio, M. A., & Moors, A. L. (2003). Evaluating mastery: Measuring instructional outcomes for children with autism. *European Journal of Behavior Analysis, 4,* 23–36.

Flick, G. L. (1998). *ADD/ADHD behavior change resource kit: Ready to use strategies and activities for helping children with attention deficit disorder.* San Francisco: Jossey-Bass.

Fombonne, E. (2003). Epidemiological surveys of autism and other pervasive developmental disorders: An update. *Journal of Autism and Developmental Disorders, 33*(4), 365–382.

Freeman, S., & Dake, L. (1997). *Teach me language: A language manual for children with autism, Asperger's syndrome and related developmental disorders.* Langley, British Columbia, Canada: SKF Books.

Frith, U., & Baron-Cohen, S. (1987). Perception in autistic children. In D. J. Cohen & A. M. Donnellan (Eds.), *Handbook of autism and pervasive developmental disorders* (pp. 85–102). New York: Wiley.

Frost, L., & Bondy, A. (1985). *The Picture Exchange Communication System.* Newark, DE: Pyramid Educational Products.

Frost, L., & Bondy, A. (2002). *The Picture Exchange Communication System* (2nd ed.). Newark, DE: Pyramid Educational Products.

Gagnon, E. (2001). *Power cards: Using special interests to motivate children and youth with Asperger syndrome and autism.* Shawnee Mission, KS: Autism Asperger.

Gallagher, T., & Prutting, C. (1983). *Pragmatic assessment and intervention issues in language.* San Diego, CA: College-Hill.

Gillberg, C. (1990). Autism and pervasive developmental disorders. *Journal of Child Psychology and Psychiatry, 31*(1), 99–119.

Gillberg, C. (1998). Asperger syndrome and high-functioning autism. *British Journal of Psychiatry, 172,* 200–209.

Goetz, L., Gee, K., & Sailor, W. (1985). Using a behavior chain interruption strategy to teach communication skills to students with severe disabilities. *Journal of the Association for Persons with Severe Handicaps, 10,* 21–30.

Goldhaber, D. (1986). *Life-span human development.* New York: Harcourt Brace.

Goleman, D. (1996). *Emotional intelligence.* New York: Bantam Books.

Graff, R. B., Green, G., & Libby, M. E. (1998). Effects of two levels of treatment intensity on a young child with severe disabilities. *Behavioral Interventions, 13,* 21–42.

Grandin, T., & Scariano, M. (1986). *Emergence labeled autistic.* Ann Arbor.

Gravel, J. S. (1994). Auditory integration training: Placing the burden of proof. *American Journal of Speech–Language Pathology, 3*(2), 25–29.

Gray, C. (2004). Social stories 10.0: The new defining criteria and guidelines. *Jenison Autism Journal, 15*(4), 2–20.

Gresham, F. M., & MacMillan, D. L. (1998). Early intervention project: Can its claims be substantiated and its effects replicated? *Journal of Autism and Developmental Disorders, 28*(1), 5–13.

Gutstein, S. E., & Sheely, R. K. (2002). *Relationship development intervention with young children.* London: Kingsley.

Harris, J. R., & Liebert, R. M. (1987). *The child: Development from birth through adolescence.* London: Prentice Hall.

Harris, S. I. (2003). Treatment of family problems in autism. In E. Schopler & G. Mesibov (Eds.), *Behavioral issues in autism* (pp. 161–175). New York: Springer.

Hart, S., Jones, N. A., & Field, T. (2003). Atypical expressions of jealousy in infants of intrusive- and withdrawn-depressed mothers. *Child Psychiatry and Human Development, 33*(3), 193–207.

Hoagwood, K., Burns, B. J., Kiser, L., Ringeisen, H., & Schoenwald, S. K. (2001). Evidence-based practice in child and adolescent mental health services. *Psychiatric Services, 52,* 1179–1189.

Hodgdon, L. A. (2000). *Visual strategies for improving communication: Practical supports for school and home.* Troy, MI: QuirkRoberts.

Horner, R. H. (2000). Positive behavior supports. *Focus on Autism and Other Developmental Disabilities, 15*(2), 97–105.

Howlin, P. (1997). Prognosis is autism: Do specialists' treatment affect long-term outcome? *European Child and Adolescent Psychiatry, 6,* 55–72.

Howlin, P., Baron-Cohen, S., & Hadwin, J. (2002). *Teaching children with autism to mind-read.* London: Kingsley.

Iwata, B., Dorsey, M. F., Slifer, K. J., Baum, K. B., & Richman, G. S. (1982). Toward a functional analysis of self-injury. *Analysis and Intervention in Develomental Disabilities, 2,* 3–20.

Johnson, K. R., & Layng, T. V. J. (1992). Breaking the structuralist barrier: Literacy and numeracy with fluency. *American Psychologist, 47,* 1475–1490.

Johnson, K., & Street, E. M. (2004). *The Morningside model of generative instruction: What it means to leave no child behind.* Concord, MA: Cambridge Center for Behavioral Studies.

Johnson-Martin, N. M. Jens, K. G., Attermeier, S. M.; & Hacker, M. H. S. (1990). *The Carolina curriculum for preschoolers with special needs.* Baltimore: Brookes.

Kanner, L. (1943). Autistic disturbances of affective contact. *Nervous Child, 2,* 217–250.

Kasari, C. (2004). Teaching joint attention and play skills to young children with autism. *Autism News of Orange County & the Rest of the World, 1*(3), 4–7.

Kasari, C., Sigman, M., & Yirmiya, N. (1993). Focused and social attention in interactions with familiar and unfamiliar adults: A comparison of autistic, mentally retarded and normal children. *Development and Psychopathology, 5,* 401–412.

Kaufman, A. S. (1994). *Intelligent testing with the WISC III.* Hoboken, NJ: Wiley.

Kerr, S., & Durkin, K. (2004). Understanding of thought bubbles as mental representations in children with autism: Implications for theory of mind. *Journal of Autism & Developmental Disorders, 34*(6), 637–648.

Kiernan, C. (1981). A strategy for research and the use of nonvocal systems of communication. *Journal of Autism and Developmental Disorders, 11,* 139–152.

Kiphard, E. J. (1996). *Wie weit ist ein Kind entwickelt?* Dortmund, Germany: Verlag Modernes Lernen.

Klicpera, C., Bormann-Kischkel, C., & Gasteiger-Klicpera, B. (2001). Autismus. In H.-C. Steinhausen (Ed.), *Entwicklungsstörungen im Kindes- und Jugendalter* (pp. 197–215). Stuttgart, Germany: Kohlhammer.

Klin, A. (2006). Autism and Asperger syndrome: An overview. *Review Brazilian Psiquiatrique, 28,* 3–11.

Koegel, L., Koegel, R., & Dunlap, G. (1996). *Positive behavioral support.* Baltimore: Brookes.

Koegel, R. L. (1999). Pivotal response intervention: Overview of approach. *Journal of the Association for the Severely Handicapped, 24,* 174–185.

Koegel, R., Camarata, S., Koegel, L., Ben-Tall, A., & Smith, A. (1998). Increasing speech intelligibility in children with autism. *Journal of Autism and Developmental Disorders, 28,* 241–251.

Koegel, R. L., & Frea, W. D. (1993). Treatment of social behavior in autism through the modification of pivotal social skills. *Journal of Applied Behavior Analysis, 26*(3), 369–377.

Koegel, R. L., & Kern-Koegel, L. (2005). *Pivotal response treatments for autism communication, social, and academic development.* Baltimore: Brookes.

Koegel, R. L., & Koegel, L. K. (1988). Generalized responsivity and pivotal behaviors. In R. Horner, G. Dunlap, & R. Koegel (Eds.), *Generalization and life-style changes in applied settings* (pp. 41–66). Baltimore: Brookes.

Koegel, R. L., O'Dell, M., & Dunlap, G. (1988). Producing speech use in non-verbal autistic children by reinforcing attempts. *Journal of Autism and Developmental Disorders, 18,* 525–538.

Koegel, R. L., Rincover, A., & Egel, A. C. (1982). *Educating and understanding autistic children.* San Diego, CA: College Hill Press.

Koegel, R., Russo, D., & Rincover, A. (1977). Assessing and training teachers in the generalized use of behavior modification with autistic children. *Journal of Applied Behavior Analysis, 10,* 197–205.

Koegel, R. L., & Williams, J. (1980). Direct versus indirect response-reinforcer relationships in teaching autistic children. *Journal of Abnormal Child Psychology, 4,* 537–547.

Kok, A., Bernard-Opitz, V., & Tan, Y. K. A. (2002). Comparison of the effects of structured and facilitated play on preschool children with autism. *Autism: The International Journal of Research and Practice, 6*(1), 181–196.

Kubina, R. M., Morrison, R., & Lee, D. L. (2002). Benefits of adding precision teaching to behavioral interventions for students with autism. *Behavioral Interventions, 17,* 233–246.

Laski, K. E., Charlop, M. H., & Schreibman, L. (1988). Training parents to use the natural language paradigm to increase their autistic children's speech. *Applied Behavior Analysis, 21*(4), 391–400.

LaVigna, G. (1977). Communication training in mute autistic adolescents using the written word. *Journal of Autism and Childhood Schizophrenia, 7,* 135–149.

Leach, D., Coyle, C. A., & Cole, P. G. (2003). Fluency in the classroom. In R. F. Waugh (Ed.), *On the forefront of educational psychology* (pp. 115–137). New York: Nova Science.

Leaf, R. (1998, February). *Evolution of behavioral treatment.* Seminar presented at the Indiana Resource Center for Autism Symposium, *Educational choices for young children with autism,* Indianapolis, IN.

Leaf, R., & McEachin, J. (1999). *A work in progress: Behavior management strategies and a curriculum for intensive behavioral treatment of autism.* New York: DLR Books.

Leroy, G., Chuang, S., Huang, J., & Charlop-Christy, M. H. (2005). Digital libraries on handhelds for autistic children. In *Proceedings of the 5th ACM/IEEE joint conference on digital libraries* (p. 387). New York: Association of Computer Machinery.

Lindsley, O. R. (1964). Direct measurement and prothesis of retarded behavior. *Journal of Education, 147,* 62–81.

Lindsley, O. R. (1972). From Skinner to precision teaching: The child knows best. In J. B. Jordan & L. S. Robbins (Eds.), *Let's try doing something else kind of thing.* Arlington, VA: Council for Exceptional Children.

Lindsley, O. R. (1990). Precision teaching: By children for teachers. *Teaching Exceptional Children, 22*(3), 10–15.

Lord, C., Rutter, M., & Le Couteur, A. (1994). Autism Diagnostic Interview–Revised: A revised version of a diagnostic interview for caregivers of individuals with possible pervasive developmental disorders. *Journal of Autism and Developmental Disorders, 24*(5), 659–685.

Lord, C., & Schopler, E. (1994). TEACCH services for preschool children. In S. L. Harris & J. S. Handleman (Eds.), *Preschool education programs for children with autism* (pp. 87–106). Austin, TX: PRO-ED.

Lovaas, O. I. (1968). A program for the establishment of speech in psychotic children. In H. N. Sloane & B. D. MacAulay (Eds.), *Operant procedures in remedial speech and language training.* Boston: Houghton Mifflin.

Lovaas, O. I. (1981). *Teaching developmentally disabled children: The Me Book.* Austin, TX: PRO-ED.

Lovaas, O. I. (1987). Behavioral treatment and normal educational and intellectual functioning in young autistic children. *Journal of Consulting and Clinical Psychology, 55,* 3–9.

Lowe, M., & Costello, A. (1988). *The Symbolic Play Test* (2nd ed.). Windsor, United Kingdom: NferNelson.

MacDuff, G. S., Krantz, P. J., & McClannahan, L. E. (1993). Teaching children with autism to use photographic activity schedules. *Journal of Applied Behavior Analysis, 26,* 89–97.

Mastergeorge, A., Rogers, S., Corbett, B., & Solomon, M. (2003). Nonmedical interventions for autism spectrum disorders. In S. Ozonoff, S. J. Rogers, & R. L. Hendren, (Eds.), *Autism spectrum disorders: A research review for practitioners* (pp. 130–160). Washington, DC: American Psychiatric.

Maurice, C., Green, G., & Luce, S. C. (1996). *Behavioral intervention for young children with autism.* Austin, TX: PRO-ED.

McClannahan, L. E., & Krantz, P. J. (1999). *Activity schedules for children with autism: Teaching independent behavior.* Bethesda, MD: Woodbine House.

McCracken, H., & Wolfberg, P. (2005). Pathways to friendship and play for children on the autism spectrum. *Autism News of Orange County and the Rest of the World, 2*(3), 4–7.

McDougle, C. J., Holmes, J. P., Carlson, D. C., Pelton, G. H., Cohen, D. J., & Price, L. H. (1998). A double-blind, placebo-controlled study of risperidone in adults with autistic disorder and other pervasive developmental disorders. *Archives of General Psychiatry, 55,* 633–641.

McEachin, J. J., Smith, T., & Lovaas, O. I. (1993). Long-term outcome for children with autism who received early intensive behavioral treatment. *American Journal on Mental Retardation, 97,* 359–372.

McKinnon, K., & Krempa, J. (2002). *Social skills solutions: A hands-on manual for teaching social skills to children with autism.* New York: DRL Books.

Mesibov, G. B., (1997). Formal and informal measures on the effectiveness of the TEACCH programme. *Autism, 1*(1) 25–35.

Mesibov, G., & Howley, M. (2003). *Assessing the curriculum for pupils with autistic spectrum disorders.* London: Fulton.

Mesibov, G. B., Schopler, E., & Hearsay, K. (1994). Structured teaching in the TEACCH system. In E. Schopler & G. B. Mesibov (Eds.), *Behavioral issues in autism* (pp. 195–207). New York: Plenum.

Mesibov, G. B., Shea, V., & Schopler, E. (2004). *The TEACCH approach to autism spectrum disorders.* New York: Springer.

Mundy, P., & Crowson, M. (1997). Joint attention and early social communication: Implications for research on intervention with autism. *Journal of Autism and Developmental Disorders, 27*(6), 653–676.

Mundy, P., Sigman, M., & Kasari, C. (1994). Joint attention, developmental level and symptom presentation in autism. *Development and Psychopathology, 6,* 389–401.

Myles, B. S., & Schapman, A. (2004). Making sense of the 'hidden curriculum.' *Autism News of Orange County and the Rest of the World, 1*(3), 16–18.

Myles, B. S., Tapscott-Cook, K., Miller, N. E., Rinner, L., & Robbins, L. (2000). *Asperger syndrome and sensory issues: Practical solutions for making sense of the world.* Shawnee Mission, KS: Autism Asperger.

Nah, Y. H. (2000). Evaluating the effectiveness of using multi-media social stories in teaching social and behavioral skills. *Autism News Singapore, 1,* 10.

National Institute of Mental Health. (2004). *Autism spectrum disorders (Pervasive developmental disorders)* (NIH Publication No. NIH.04-5511). Bethesda, MD: Author.

Panarai, S., Ferrante, L., & Zingale, M. (2002). Benefits of the treatment and education of autistic and communicatively handicapped children (TEACCH) programme as compared with a non-specific approach. *Journal of Intellectual Disability Research, 46*(4), 318–327.

Partington, J. W., & Sundberg, M. L. (1998). *The assessment of basic language and learning skills.* Pleasant Hill, CA: Behavior Analysts.

Payne, P. C. (2003). *LINKS to language.* Workshop sponsored by the Orange County Department of Education, Irvine, CA.

Pennypacker, H. S., Koenig, C. H., & Lindsley, O. R. (1972). *Handbook of the standard behavior chart.* Kansas City, KS: Precision Media.

Perry, A., & Condillac, R. (2003). *Evidence-based practices for children and adolescents with autism spectrum disorders: Review of the literature and practice guide.* Toronto, Ontario, Canada: Children's Mental Health Ontario.

Piaget, J. (1962). *Play, dreams and imitation in childhood.* New York: Norton.

Pretti-Frontczak, K., & Bricker, D. (2004). *An activity-based approach to early intervention* (3rd ed.). Baltimore: Brookes.

Prior, R., & Cummins, M. (1992). Questions about facilitated communication and autism. *Journal of Autism and Developmental Disorders, 22,* 331.

Prizant, B. M., Schuler, A. L. Wetherby, A. M., & Rydell, P. (1997). Enhancing language and communication: Language approaches. In D. Cohen & F. Volkmar (Eds.), *Handbook of autism and pervasive developmental disorders* (2nd ed.). New York: Wiley.

Prizant, B. M., & Wetherby, A. M. (1998). Understanding the continuum of discrete-trial traditional behavioral to social-pragmatic developmental approaches in communication enhancement for young children with autism/PDD. *Seminars in Speech and Language, 19*(4), 329–353.

Prizant, M. B., Wetherby, A. M., Rubin, E., Laurent, A. C., & Rydell, P. J. (2005). *The SCERTS model: A comprehensive educational approach for children with autism spectrum disorders.* Baltimore: Brookes.

Quill, K. A. (2002). *Do, watch, listen, say.* Baltimore: Brookes.

Raven, J. C. (2004). *Progressive matrices.* Orlando, FL: Harcourt Assessment.

Rincover, A. (1978). Sensory extinction: A procedure for eliminating self-stimulatory behavior in developmentally disabled children. *Journal of Abnormal Child Psychology, 6,* 299–310.

Rincover, A., Cook, R., Peoples, A., & Packard, D. (1979). Sensory extinction and sensory reinforcement principles for programming multiple adaptive behavior change. *Journal of Applied Behaviour Analysis, 12*(2), 221–233.

Rodrigue, J. R., Morgan, S. B., & Geffken, G. R. (1990). Families of autistic children: Psychosocial functioning of mothers. *Journal of Clinical Child Psychology, 19,* 371–379.

Roid, G., & Miller, L. (1997). *Leiter International Performance Scale-Revised Edition*. Wood Dale, IL: Stoelting.

Salisch, M. (2002). *Emotionale Kompetenz entwickeln*. Stuttgart, Germany: Kohlhammer Verlag.

Sallows, G. O., & Graupner, T. D. (1999, May). *Replicating Lovaas' treatment and findings: Preliminary results*. Paper presented at PEACH Conference, London.

Schopler, E., Lansing, M. D., & Waters, L. (1982). *Teaching activities for autistic children: Vol. III. Individualized assessment and treatment for autistic and developmentally disabled children*. Austin, TX: PRO-ED.

Schopler, E., Lansing, M., & Waters, L. (1983). *Individualized assessment and treatment for autistic and developmentally disabled children*. Baltimore: University Park Press.

Schopler, E., & Mesibov, G. (1994). *Behavioral issues in autism*. New York: Plenum.

Schopler, E., Mesibov, G. B., & Shea, V. (2004). *The TEACCH approach to autism spectrum disorders*. New York: Plenum.

Schopler, E., Reichler, R. J., Bashford, A., Lansing, M. D., & Marcus, L. M. (1990). *Psychoeducational Profile–Revised*. Austin, TX: PRO-ED.

Schreibman, L., & Carr, E. G. (1978). Elimination of echolalic responding to questions through the training of a generalized verbal response. *Journal of Applied Behavior Analysis, 11*(4), 453–463.

Schreibman, L., & Koegel, R. L. (2005). Training for parents of children with autism: Pivotal responses, generalization, and individualization of interventions. In E. D. Hibbs & P. S. Jensen (Eds.), *Psychosocial treatment for child and adolescent disorders: Empirically based strategies for clinical practice* (2nd ed., pp. 605–631). Washington, DC: American Psychological Association.

Schuler, A. L. (1989). The assessment of communicative competence. Seminars in Speech and Language, American Speech-Hearing-Language Association.

Schuler, A. L., & Wolfberg, P. (2000). Promoting peer play and socialization: The art of scaffolding. In A. Wetherby & B. M. Prizant (Eds.), *Transactional foundations of language intervention*. Baltimore: Brookes.

Schwaab, D. (1992). Bilder und Zeichnungen autistisch Behinderter: Ihre Funktion in der Entwicklung und Biologie. Dorothea Schwaab Stiftung (Ed.), *Neustadt an der Weinstrasse:* Birghan.

Seligman, M. (1975). *Helplessness: Depression, development and death*. New York: Freeman.

Shane, H. C. (1994). *Facilitated communication: The clinical and social phenomenon*. San Diego, CA: Singular.

Shaw, S. R. (2002). A school psychologist investigates sensory integration therapies: Promise, possibility, and the art of placebo. *NASP Communiqué*.

Shea, V. (2004). A perspective on the research literature related to early intensive behavioral intervention (Lovaas) for young children with autism. *The International Journal of Research & Practice: Autism, 8*(4), 349–367.

Sherer M. R., & Schreibman, L. (2005). Individual behavioral profiles and predictors of treatment effectiveness for children with autism. *Journal of Consulting & Clinical Psychology, 73*(3), 525–538.

Shure, M. B. (2003). *I can problem solve: An interpersonal cognitive problem-solving program*. Champaign, IL: Research Press.

Siegel, B. (2003). *Helping children with autism learn: Treatment approaches for parents and professionals*. Oxford, England: Oxford University Press.

Sigman, M., & Ungerer, J. (1984). Cognitive and language skills in autistic, mentally retarded, and normal children. *Developmental Psychology, 20*, 293–302.

Silver Lining Multimedia. (2003). *Picture This* [Computer software]. Peterborough, NH: Author.

Simmons, E. K., Derby, M., & McLaughlin, T. F. (1998). The use of functional communication training and precision teaching to reduce the challenging behavior of a toddler with autism. *Journal of Precision Teaching and Celeration, 13*(2), 50–55.

Sparrow, S., Balla, D., & Cicchetti, D. (1984). *Vineland Adaptive Behavior Scales*. Circle Pines, MN: American Guidance Service.

Stone, W. L., Ousley, O. Y., Yoder, P. J., Hogan, K. L., & Hepburn, S. L. (1997). Nonverbal communication in two- and three-year-old children with autism. *Journal of Autism and Developmental Disorders, 27*, 677–696.

Sundberg, M. L., & Partington, J. W. (1999). The need for both discrete trial and natural environment language training for children with autism. In P. M. Ghezzi, W. L. Williams, & J. E. Carr (Eds.), *Autism: Behavior-analytic perspectives* (pp. 139–156). Reno, NV: Context Press.

Symons, F. J., Thompson, A., & Rodriguez, M. C. (2004). Self-injurious behavior and the efficacy of naltrexone treatment: A quantitative synthesis. *Mental Retardation and Developmental Disabilities Research Reviews, 10*(3), 193–200.

Tan, Y. K., & Bernard-Opitz, V. (2002). *Teaching joint attention in young children with autism: An exploratory study*. Unpublished manuscript.

Thompson, T., Symons, F., Delaney, D., & England, C. (1995). Self-injurious behavior as endogenous neurochemical self-administration. *Mental Retardation and Developmental Disabilities Research Review, 1*(2), 137–148.

Trehin, G. (2004). Welcome to Gilles Trehin's world. *Autism News of Orange County and the Rest of the World, 1*(2), 16–17.

Twachtman-Cullen, D. (2004). Ten take-home messages for successful language intervention. *Autism News of Orange County and the Rest of the World, 1*(2), 8–9.

Van Houten, R., & Nau, P. A. (1980). A comparison of the effects of fixed and variable ratio schedules of reinforcement on the behavior of deaf children. *Journal of Applied Behavior Analysis, 13*(1), 13–21.

Vargas, E. A., & Vargas, J. S. (1991). Programmed instruction: What it is and how to do it. *Journal of Behavioral Education, 1*(2), 235–251.

Volkmar, F. R., Klin, A., & Cohen, D. J. (1997). Diagnosis and classification of autism and related conditions: Consensus issues. In D. J. Cohen & F. R. Volkmar (Eds.), *Handbook of autism and pervasive developmental disorders* (pp. 5–40). New York: Wiley.

Von Gontard, A. (2004). *Enkopresis. Erscheinungsformen–Diagnostik–Therapie.* Stuttgart, Germany: Kohlhammer.

Weiss, M. J., & Harris, S. L. (2001). *Reaching out, joining in: Teaching social skills to young children with autism.* Bethesda, MD: Woodbine House.

Wellman H. M., Baron-Cohen S., Caswell R., Gomez, J. C., Swettenham J., Toye E., et al. (2002). Thought-bubbles help children with autism acquire an alternative to a theory of mind. *Autism: The International Journal of Research & Practice, 6*(4), 343–363.

Welsh, M. (1989). *Holding time: How to eliminate conflict, temper tantrums, and sibling rivalry, and raise happy, loving, successful children.* New York: Fireside.

Wetherby, A., & Prizant, B. (1993). Profiling communication and symbolic profiles of young children. *Journal of Childhood Communicative Disorders, 15*, 23–32.

Wetherby, A., & Prutting, C. (1989). Profiles of communicative and cognitive–social abilities in autistic children. *Journal of Speech and Hearing Research, 27*, 364–377.

White, G. B., & White, M. S. (1987). Autism from the inside. *Medical Hypothesis, 24*, 223–229.

White, O. R. (1986). Precision teaching–precision learning. *Exceptional Children, 52*, 522–534.

White, O. R., & Haring, N. G. (1981). *Exceptional teaching* (2nd ed.). Columbus, OH: Merrill.

White, T., & Schultz, S. K. (2000). Naltrexone treatment for a 3-year-old boy with self-injurious behavior. *American Journal of Psychiatry, 157*, 1574–1582.

Williams, D. (1992). *Nobody nowhere.* New York: Random House.

Wing, L. (1988). The continuum of autistic disorders. In E. Schopler & G. M. Mesibov (Eds.), *Diagnosis and assessment in autism* (pp. 91–110). New York: Plenum.

Wing, L., & Gould, J. (1979). Severe impairments of social interaction and associated abnormalities in children: Epidemiology and classification. *Journal of Autism and Childhood Schizophrenia, 9*, 11–29.

Winner, M. G. (2002). *Inside out: What makes the person with Asperger syndrome tick?* San Jose, CA: Author.

Wolfberg, P. J. (2003). *Peer play and the autism spectrum: The art of guiding children's socialization and imagination.* Shawnee Mission, KS: Autism Asperger.

Wolfberg, P. J., & Schuler, A. L. (1993). Integrated play groups: A model for promoting the social and cognitive dimensions of play in children with autism. *Journal of Autism and Developmental Disorders, 23*, 467–489.

Yang, T. R., Wolfberg, P. J., & Wu, S.-C. (2003). Supporting children on the autism spectrum in peer play at home and school: Piloting the integrated playgroups model in Taiwan. *Autism: The International Journal of Research and Practice, 7*(4), 437–453.

Zercher, C., Hunt, P., Schuler, A., & Webster, J. (2001). Increasing joint attention, play, and language through peer-supported play. *Autism, 5*(4), 374–398.

Web Sites

GENERAL INFORMATION

Association for Science in Treatment of Autism
www.asatonline.org

Autism Europe
www.autismeurope.org/portal

Autism Information Center from the Centers for Disease Control and Prevention
www.cdc.gov/ncbddd/dd/ddautism.htm

Autism Institute on Peer Relations and Play
www.autisminstitute.com

Autism Society of America
www.autism-society.org

Autism Speaks
www.autismspeaks.org

California Department of Developmental Services Information on Autism
www.dds.ca.gov/autism/autism_main.cfm

Cambridge Center for Behavioral Studies
www.behavior.org

Center for the Study of Autism
www.autism.org

Division TEACCH
www.teacch.com

National Autistic Society
www.england.autism.org.uk/nas/jsp/polopoly.jsp?d=10

Princeton Child Development Institute
www.pcdi.org/aboutUs/index.asp

University of California Davis Mind Institute
www.ucdmc.ucdavis.edu/mindinstitute

World Autism Organization (links to organizations around the world)
www.worldautism.org

Yale Developmental Disabilities Clinic
info.med.yale.edu/chldstdy/autism/index.html

JOURNALS AND NEWSLETTERS

Autism Asperger's Digest Magazine
www.autismdigest.com

Autism: The International Journal of Research and Practice
www.sagepub.com/journal.aspx?pid=79

Autism News of Orange County and the Rest of the World
www.verabernard.org/news.htm

Journal of Applied Behavior Analysis
seab.envmed.rochester.edu/jaba

Journal of Autism and Developmental Disorders
www.ovid.com/site/catalog/Journal/270.jsp?top=2&mid=3&bottom=7&subsection=12

PRODUCTS

Autism Teaching Tools
www.autismteachingtools.com

Boardmaker
www.mayer-johnson.com

Do to Learn
www.do2learn.com

Future Horizons
www.futurehorizons-autism.com

Progressive Academic Learning System
www.palsprogram.com

Pyramid–Picture Exchange Communication System
www.pecs.com

Shoebox Tasks
www.shoeboxtasks.com

Silver Lining Multimedia
www.silverliningmm.com

Special Needs Project (for books and videos)
www.specialneeds.com

Tasks Galore
www.tasksgalore.com

Visual Strategies
www.usevisualstrategies.com

Glossary

Applied Behavior Analysis (ABA)   is the application of behavioral principles to the analysis of behavior. "Applied" refers to behavior, which is meaningful or functional for the individual child. ABA is widely regarded as the most researched intervention in addressing the social, linguistic, and cognitive differences in children with autism spectrum disorders.

Attention-Deficit Disorder (ADD)   is a neurologically based disturbance of attention and behavior, which sometimes is associated with hyperactivity.

Autism Spectrum Disorders (ASD) or Pervasive Developmental Disorders   range from a severe form called early infantile autism or autistic disorder to a milder form called Asperger syndrome or high-level autism. The diagnostic criteria include communication problems, ritualistic behaviors, and inappropriate social interaction.

Discrete Trial Format (DTF)   is a behavioral intervention method characterized by clear task setup, discriminative instructions, effective prompts, and consequences.

Experience-Based Learning or Activity-Based Instructions   refers to teaching methods that allow children experience in daily settings. Handling and exploring objects, using common material and activities, and providing emotional experiences are characteristic of this approach.

Natural Language Paradigm (NLP)   combines traditional behavioral methods with developmental and linguistic approaches. The child's initiative and everyday settings are crucial in interventions.

The Picture Exchange Communication System (PECS)   is a training program aimed especially at nonverbal children. Children learn to communicate requests through exchanging pictures for the real items. At a later stage, other communicative functions can be taught.

Pivotal Response Training (PRT)   is a behavioral method that stresses the child's initiative in learning. Motivation is enhanced through providing choices, reinforcing the child's attempts to communicate, and using natural reinforcers.

Precision Teaching (PT) or Fluency Learning   aims at automatic responding of mastered behavior. Teaching targets are broken down into small learning slices, which are practiced within small time units of 10, 20, 30, or 60 seconds.

Structured Therapy (ST)   refers to teaching methods that are based on empirical evidence. They have a clear structure and a direct link to the problems of children with ASD.

Structured Therapy and Experience-Based Programs (STEP)   include the following teaching methods: discrete trial format, precision teaching, experience-based methods, and visual systems.

Treatment and Education for Autistic and Related Communication Handicapped Children Program (TEACCH)   is an intervention system that originated at the University of North Carolina and has affected autism programs throughout the world. Characteristic features are visual support, clear learning structures, and independence.

Subject Index

About the Author

Vera Bernard-Opitz, PhD, has worked as a clinical psychologist and behavior therapist with more than 1,000 children with autism spectrum disorders (ASD) in autism centers, schools, and behavioral research centers in the United States, Germany, and Singapore. As associate professor at the National University of Singapore, she initiated and coordinated structured teaching programs for children with ASD for 15 years. She has published several books and has contributed various articles in international journals. She presently is the editor of the *Autism News of Orange County and the Rest of the World,* an autism newsletter. She works as an international consultant, giving workshops and providing video consultations to help children with autism around the globe. Her Web site can be found at www.verabernard.org.